Walid FEKI
Rim KAMMOUN
Khouloud AbdelMouleh

Indicators of the severity of bronchial dilatation

Walid FEKI
Rim KAMMOUN
Khouloud AbdelMouleh

Indicators of the severity of bronchial dilatation

ScienciaScripts

Imprint
Any brand names and product names mentioned in this book are subject to trademark, brand or patent protection and are trademarks or registered trademarks of their respective holders. The use of brand names, product names, common names, trade names, product descriptions etc. even without a particular marking in this work is in no way to be construed to mean that such names may be regarded as unrestricted in respect of trademark and brand protection legislation and could thus be used by anyone.

Cover image: www.ingimage.com

This book is a translation from the original published under ISBN 978-620-6-71074-5.

Publisher:
Sciencia Scripts
is a trademark of
Dodo Books Indian Ocean Ltd. and OmniScriptum S.R.L publishing group

120 High Road, East Finchley, London, N2 9ED, United Kingdom
Str. Armeneasca 28/1, office 1, Chisinau MD-2012, Republic of Moldova, Europe
Managing Directors: Ieva Konstantinova, Victoria Ursu
info@omniscriptum.com

Printed at: see last page
ISBN: 978-620-8-56434-6

Contents

Introduction

Bronchial dilatation (BDB) or bronchiectasis is a chronic disabling respiratory pathology characterised by irreversible dilatation of the small and medium-calibre bronchial lumen located between the 4th and 8th orders of division (1).

Although DDB has been considered an under-diagnosed condition, over the last five years its frequency has increased markedly due to the availability of high-resolution CT scans and epidemiological studies. In the UK, the prevalence in women rose from 350.5 per 100,000 population in 2004 to 566.1 in 2013, and in men from 301.2 per 100,000 population in 2004 to 485.5 per 100,000 population in 2013 (2). Global data confirm the significant morbidity and healthcare burden associated with this disorder, particularly among people with low socio-economic status. According to a recent review of the literature (3), the cost of the disease was mainly due to hospitalisations in patients with a history of repeated exacerbations.

Recurrent infections are responsible for tissue damage and inflammation, leading to the production of excess mucus and damage to the mucociliary mat. A vicious circle of COLE, tissue destruction and bronchial superinfections is then triggered (4), leading to exacerbations and, consequently, a decline in respiratory function (5,6).

To manage these patients appropriately, the clinician must first :

- Identifying highly symptomatic patients at risk of exacerbations

and those whose respiratory function has collapsed. These patients are the target of multidisciplinary management and relatively intensive therapy. Mild-risk patients, on the other hand, require simpler management and do not require specialist follow-up.

Two specific severity scores for bronchiectasis have been developed to give a better idea of the impact of the disease and thus guide the clinician's therapeutic management: bronchiectasis severity index (BSI) (7) and FACED score (8,9).

Each of the two scores assigns points for age, percentage value of forced expiratory volume in one second (FEV1), presence of colonisation by Pseudomonas Aeruginosa, radiological extension and dyspnoea stage according to the MRC scale. The BSI score also allocates points for body mass index (BMI), frequency of exacerbations, hospitalisation, and colonisation by bacteria other than Pseudomonas Aeruginosa. The scores are then calculated to classify patients into three risk groups: mild, moderate and high.

The BSI score was established following a large study in Edinburgh, UK, and subsequently validated in 4 international cohorts. The FACED score was developed specifically to predict mortality, whereas the BSI score predicts mortality, severe exacerbations and the frequency of exacerbations, and provides an estimate of quality of life (10,11,12,13).

Several parameters can influence these two scores, in particular factors specific to each population.

No study has verified the applicability of these 2 severity scores or evaluated the best score for our population.

The aim of our study was to investigate any correlation that might exist between the various severity parameters and the BSI and FACED scores, and consequently to be able to choose the best score for our population.

CHAPTER I

Patients and methods

1. Type of study

This is a single-centre comparative study (Pneumology Department of the Hédi Chaker University Hospital, Sfax), covering the period from [1]January 2009 to 31 December 2018.

2. Study population

2.1. Inclusion criteria

- Age > 16
- Bronchial dilatation confirmed by a thoracic CT scan

2.2. Non-inclusion criteria

Patients with cystic fibrosis.

Dilatation of the bronchi accompanying other pathologies, in particular pulmonary fibrosis and bronchopulmonary cancer.

3. Data collection

We consulted the medical records of the patients selected and collected a number of clinical, para-clinical and therapeutic data.

A chart analysis grid was drawn up for each patient in order obtain data that was as homogeneous as possible (Appendix 1).

Elements of the interview

- Age
- Sex
- Personal history
- Family history of neoplasia
- Lifestyle habits
- Functional respiratory, extra-respiratory and general signs. Haemoptysis was sought in all patients. Severity was assessed on the basis of the volume of bleeding observed, the underlying condition (subjacent respiratory insufficiency) and the impact on respiratory and haemodynamic status.

3.1 . Data from the clinical examination

- The patient's general condition (Organisation for Economic Co-operation and Development performance status index).

World Health Organization)

- Respiratory status :

o Presence of bronchial rales, crackles and even sibilants on auscultation, indicating bronchial congestion.

o Digital hippocratism, which may indicate progressive respiratory failure.

Extra-respiratory signs: signs of right heart failure, sinusitis which may be of value in orienting the diagnosis.

3.2 . Additional examinations

3.2.1. Imaging

Chest X-ray

It is often pathological and reveals two types of anomaly.

Direct anomalies

J Tubular walls: these are the spontaneous visibility of the thickened bronchial walls through the uncondensed parenchyma.

J Annular clefts (areolar images): Same thing seen in section

J V" or "Y" shaped tubular opacities: correspond to bronchial tubes

The bronchial tubes are solid and oriented along the axis of the bronchi. They are reflected by mucoid impactions with a parahilar distribution and a lobar bronchocele.

J Rosette or "pseudo-honeycomb" appearance: this is the result of cylindrical or varicose bronchiectasis, juxtaposed one against the other and viewed in transverse section.

J Multi-cavity appearance within which there may be fluid levels. This is the radiological translation of saccular or cystic bronchiectasis.

Indirect anomalies

J Images of atelectasis and uni or multi-lobar collapse

Chest scan

The thoracic CT scan was of great value in our study. It was requested in fine, millimetre slices and made it possible to :

- Demonstrate bronchial dilatation in any of the following situations:

J the intra-bronchial diameter is greater than that of the satellite artery

J the bronchial tubes are visualised in the outer 1/3 of the lung parenchyma

J absence of progressive reduction in bronchial calibre as you move away from the hilum.

- Determine the type of bronchial dilatation: cylindrical, moniliform, cystic according to Reid's classification.
- Assessing the extent of DDB
- Specify any complications.

3.2.2. Spirometry

Spirometry was used to measure the patients' respiratory function and therefore to determine the type of respiratory functional abnormality and its degree of severity. Spirometry was not performed on patients with medical contraindications.

3.2.3. Cytobacteriological examination of sputum

Cytobacteriological examination of the sputum was used to detect the type of infection or colonisation, which may be an indirect sign of severity. Bacterial colonisation was defined according to Spanish recommendations(14) by the presence of the same germ in 2 sputum samples taken within the previous year and at least 3 months apart.

3.3 Severity scores

Charlson comorbidity index (CCI)

This score has been used study comorbidities and predict short- and long-term survival (15). The score is made up of 19 comorbidity categories (Appendix 2). Each disease is weighted differently according to the strength of its association with one-year mortality. The total CCI score is calculated by summing the weights associated with each comorbid condition presented by the patient. Higher scores indicate more severe disorders and, consequently, a poorer prognosis.

BSI score

This score includes 9 variables (Appendix 3). The total score corresponds to the sum of the scores for each variable and varies between 0 and 26 points. Based on the total score, patients will be classified into 3 groups: low BSI score (0-4 points), intermediate BSI score (5-8 points), high BSI score (> 9).

FACED score

This score includes 5 dichotomous variables (Appendix 4). The total score corresponds to the sum of the scores for each variable and varies between 0 and 7 points.

It is used to classify DDB into 3 risk groups: mild DDB (0-2 points), moderate DDB (3-4 points) and severe DDB (5-7 points).

Estimation of quality of life

***The St Georges Respiratory Questionnaire (SGRQ)**

This score has been validated for certain respiratory diseases such as chronic obstructive pulmonary disease (COPD) and asthma. It has been validated in DDB and translated into several languages(16,17). The SGRQ comprises 50 items divided into 3 dimensions: symptoms, activity and impact on professional activity, daily life and emotional impact. A score ranging from 0 to 100 is given for each dimension, as is the total score (Appendix 5).

***HAD scale (Hospital Anxiety And Depression scale)**

This scale is used to screen for anxiety and depressive disorders. It comprises 14 items rated from 0 to 3. Seven questions relate to anxiety (total A) and seven others to depression (total D), giving 2 scores. For each dimension, a score between 0 and 7 means no symptoms, between 8 and 10 means doubtful symptoms and at from 11 onwards means definite symptoms. If we consider the two dimensions together, a score greater than or equal to 15 is a score in favour of anxiety-depressive disorders. (Appendix 6)

3.4 Therapeutics used

The type of treatment was assessed by the investigating doctor. The more severe the disease, the more intense the treatment.

3.5 Evolution and survival

For the survival and evolution, we have referred to the patients when they contained information information. For patients, we tried to contact them or their parents by post or telephone.

4. Statistical study

The data were entered and analysed using SPSS II version 20 software. Numerical values expressed as mean plus or minus standard deviation. The association between qualitative variables was calculated using Fisher's corrected Chi2 test for small numbers. Comparisons between quantitative variables were made using Student's T test. Significance is acquired for a $p < 0.05$ for all statistical tests.

CHAPTER II

Results

1. Study of the overall population

1.1.Epidemiology

1.1.1. Incidence

We collected 110 cases. The overall characteristics of the patients followed were summarised in Table II. To calculate the severity scores and throughout the prognostic part of the study, we excluded 8 patients who did not have a spirometry because of non-cooperation.

Sex

The population was characterised by a sex ratio of 1.4, i.e. 64 men (58%) and 46 women (42%) (Figure 1).

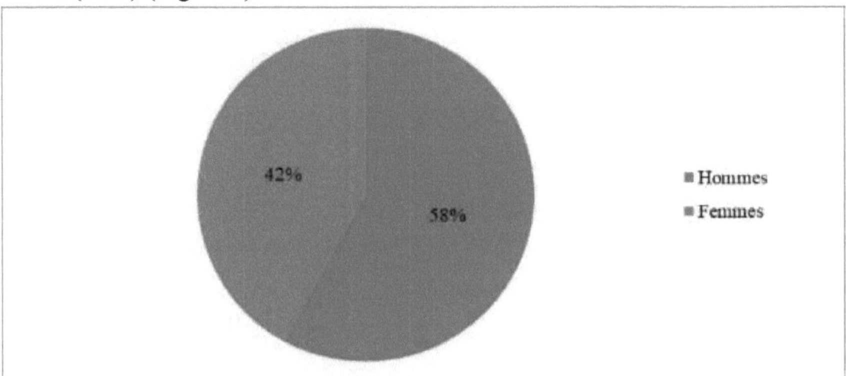

Figure 1: Breakdown of patients by gender

1.1.2. Age

The average age of patients was 60, ranging from 16 to 90, with a peak in the over-70 age group (Figure 2).

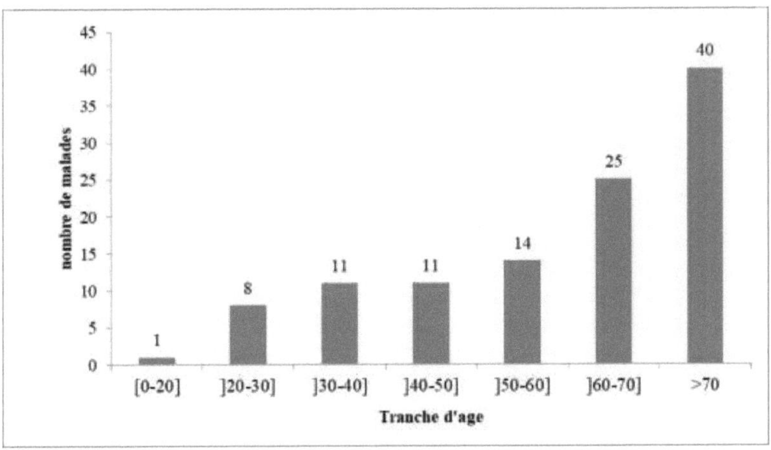

Figure 2: Breakdown of patients by age group

1.1.3. Habits

1.1.3.1. Smoking

We identified 50 active smokers in our population, 95% of whom were men. The average number of packets smoked per year was 26. Smoking cessation was achieved in 24 patients.

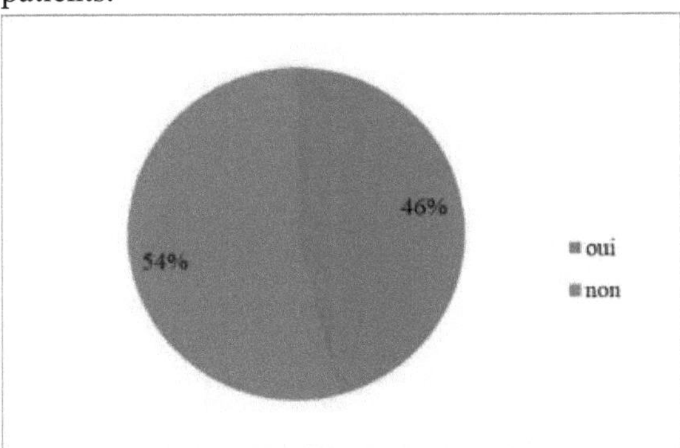

Figure 3: Percentage of the population who smoke

1.1.3.2. Alcoholism

Our population included 3 alcoholics, 2 of whom were at the stage of liver cirrhosis.

1.1.4. Personal history

A personal medical history found in 92 patients, i.e. 84% of cases. Gastro resophageal reflux disease (GERD) and arterial hypertension predominated. Body mass index was calculated for all patients, with an average BMI of 23.39, ranging from 13 to 38.

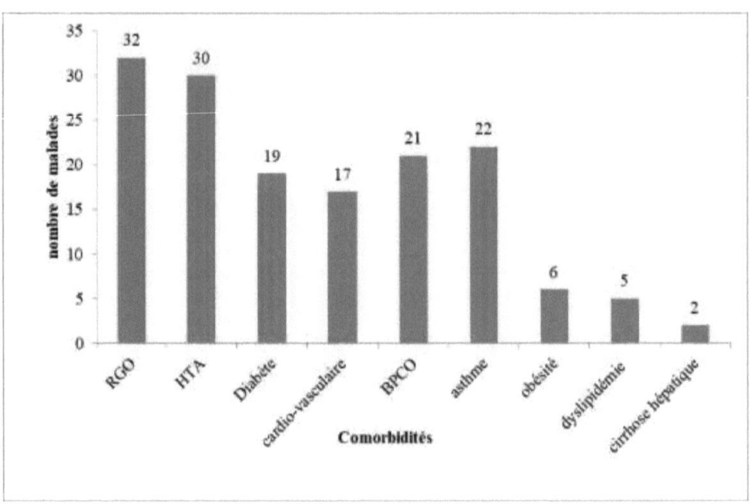

Figure 4: Breakdown of patients' personal medical history

The Charlson score (CCI) was calculated for all patients. Thirteen patients had a CCI of 0, the majority of patients had a score between 1 and 4 (66%) (Figure 5).

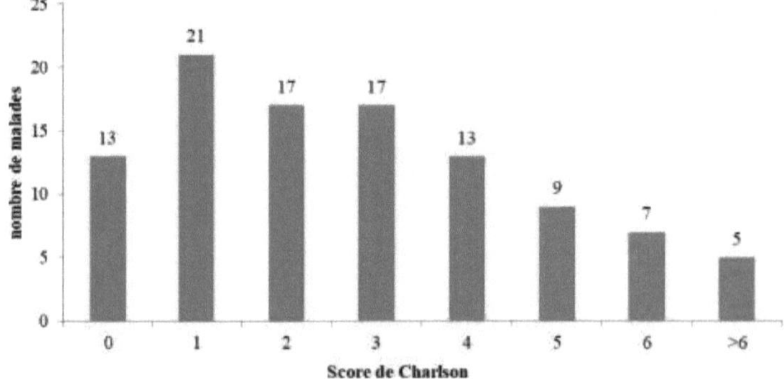

Figure 5: Distribution of patients according to Charlson score

1.1.5. Socio-economic level

We divided the population into 3 categories according to patients' socio-economic level, based in particular on profession, home town and living conditions.

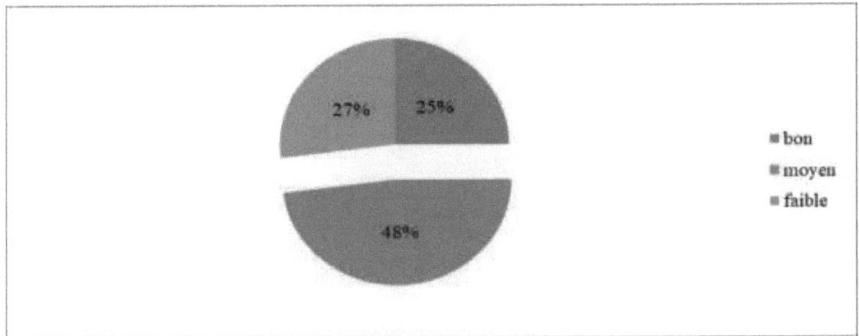

Figure 6: Breakdown of patients by socio-economic status

1.2.Clinical study

Functional respiratory signs

We investigated the main respiratory symptoms of DDB on questioning: exertional dyspnoea, haemoptysis and morning bronchorrhoea. Other clinical signs included chronic cough, particularly productive cough, chest pain and recurrent lower respiratory infections (Figure 7).

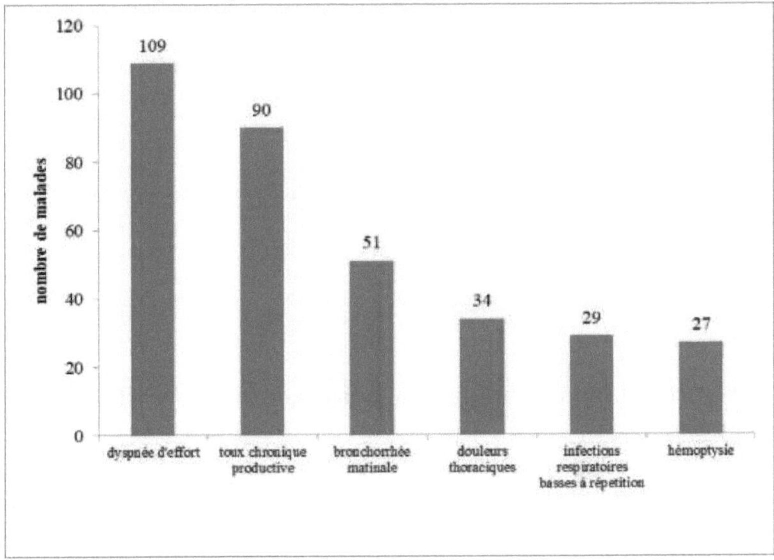

Figure 7: Symptoms of DDB

Dyspnoea on exertion :

Dyspnoea on exertion was the most frequent clinical sign. Using the MRC classification, we found that the majority of our population were at stage 3 (Figure 8).

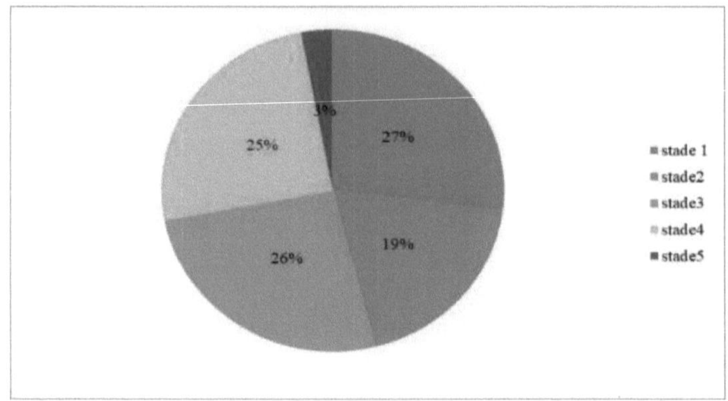

Figure 8: Distribution of patients according to exertional dyspnoea

Productive cough :

With regard to productive cough, we found that the colour of sputum, outside episodes of exacerbation, was highly variable. (Figure 9)

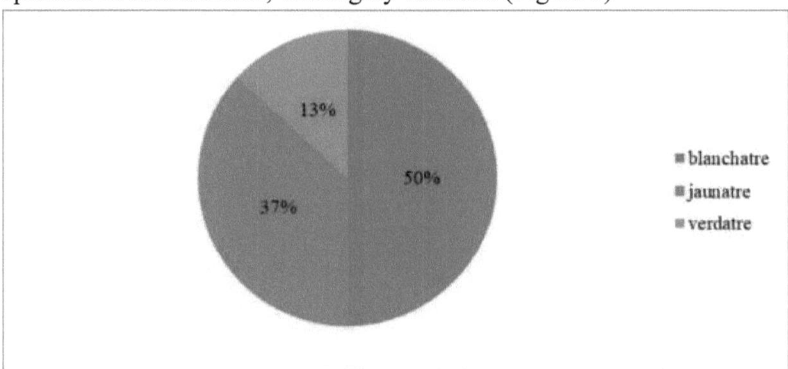

Figure 9: Colour of sputum in patients outside exacerbations

Haemoptysis :

In all cases of haemoptysis, we looked for signs of severity and assessed the volume. Severe haemoptysis requiring emergency embolisation was diagnosed in 2 patients. Recurrence of haemoptysis occurred in 16 cases.

Physical examination :

Apart from infectious outbreaks, the physical examination was normal in 85% of cases. Chest auscultation abnormalities were dominated by grumbling bronchial rales. Digital hippocratism was observed in 15 patients, more frequently in extensive and long-standing forms.

1.3.Paraclinical study

1.3.1 Thoracic imaging

1.3.1.1 Standard chest X-ray

Chest radiography was performed in all patients, with pathological findings in 95% of cases. We looked for direct abnormalities, particularly tubular cloudiness (30%), annular cloudiness (25%) and multi-cavity images (45%) (Figure 10).

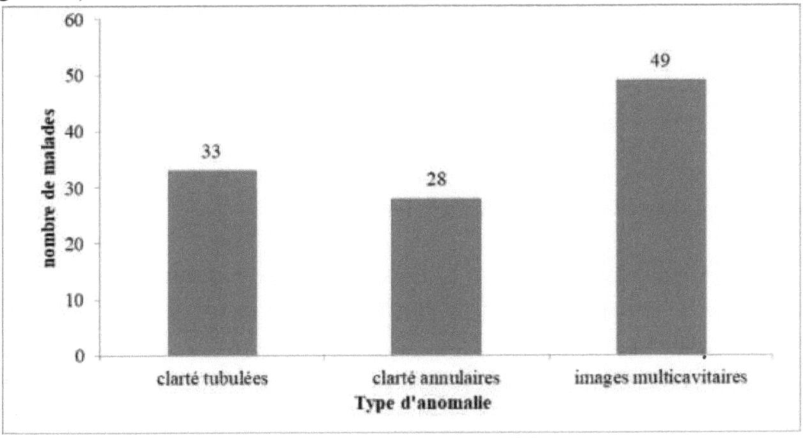

Figure 10: Description of chest X-ray abnormalities

We studied the topography and type of lesions on thoracic CT. Lesions predominated in 2 lobes (38%). The average number of lobes affected was 3.27.

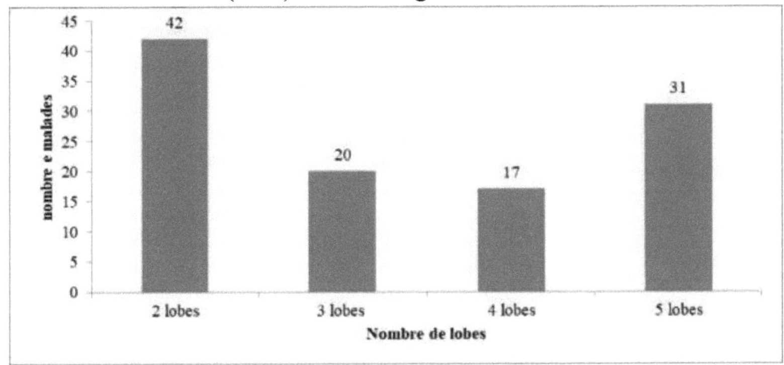

Figure 11: Number of lobes affected in our population

Cylindrical forms were the most common in our population, followed by cystic and moniliform forms (Figure 12). Associations between the 3 types were observed in 51.9% of cases. Emphysema was present in 30.4% of cases.

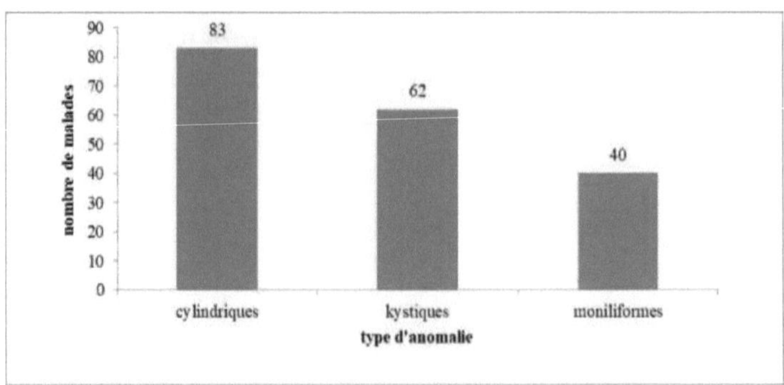

Figure 12: Types of lesions on thoracic CT scan

Other associated disorders such as mediastino-hilar adenopathies were frequent (32%). They were predominantly mediastinal (91%). Associated pleurisy was diagnosed in 4 cases.

1.3.2 Cytobacteriological examination of sputum

An ECBC was performed in all patients. Twenty-four patients were infected with Pseudomonas Aeruginosa, 5 of whom were colonised. Similarly, twenty-two patients had a history of superinfection with a germ other than pyocyanins but were not colonised by these germs.

1.3.3 Functional respiratory investigation

The mean value of FEV1 was 52%, with extremes ranging from 17% to 93%, and we divided our population into 4 groups according to the percentage value of FEV1 (Table 1). An obstructive ventilatory disorder was found in 49 cases and a restrictive disorder to a lesser extent in 30 cases.

Table I: Distribution of patients according to FEV1

Group	FEV1	(n)	%	
light	>80	8		7
Moderate	50-80	53	48	
Severe	30-49	34	31	
very severe	<30	15	14	
Total		**110**		

Table II: General characteristics of patients in our population

Patient characteristics	
Gender	46 ? ; 64 J
Average age (years)	60
BMI (average)	23,39
Dyspnoea MRC (median)	3

FEV1 (%)	52%
Colonisation by Pseudomonas Aeruginosa	5
Colonisation by other germs	0
Number of lobes affected (average)	3
Exacerbation in previous year (average)	2
Hospitalisation in the previous 2 years (average)	1,42

1.3.4 Etiologies of DDB

An aetiological investigation was requested for all patients. HBD of unknown origin (idiopathic) accounted for 65% of cases.

The aetiologies were characterised by their variability. Pulmonary tuberculosis was diagnosed in 21 patients (19%), and DDB secondary to severe infectious pneumopathy in childhood was found in 10 patients (9%). Similarly, a systemic disease or vasculitis was diagnosed in 8 cases, including rheumatoid arthritis (n=5), Gougerot Sjogren's syndrome (n=2) and Wegener's disease (n=1).

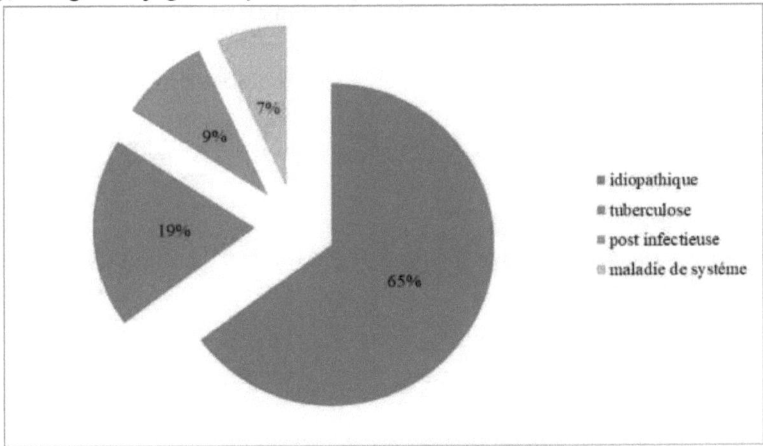

Figure 13: Etiologies of DDB

1.3.5 Treatment of DDB

Treatment for DDB has been characterised by variability in prescribing and is highly dependent on the patient's clinical signs. We have illustrated the different drugs used in DDB in Figure 14.

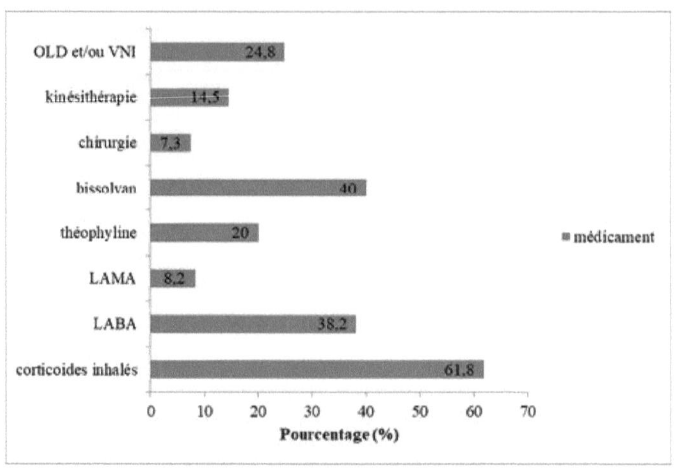

Figure 14: Drugs used in DDB

1.4 Prognostic study

In this section, we have excluded 8 patients who did not undergo spirometry (non-cooperators), thus preventing the calculation of severity scores. The total number of patients in this section will therefore be reduced to 102.

1.4.1 Mortality

1.4.1.1 Mortality rates

Twenty-one patients had died at the time of the study. The mortality rate was therefore 20.6%.

1.4.1.2 Prognostic factors :

1.4.1.2.1 Age :

The average age of patients who died was 69±17.6 years and that of survivors was 57.6±17.59 years, with a statistically significant difference (p=0.009). Mortality increased with age, rising from 2% in patients aged under 40 to 4.9% between 40 and 65 and 13.7% in patients aged over 65. The difference is not statistically significant.

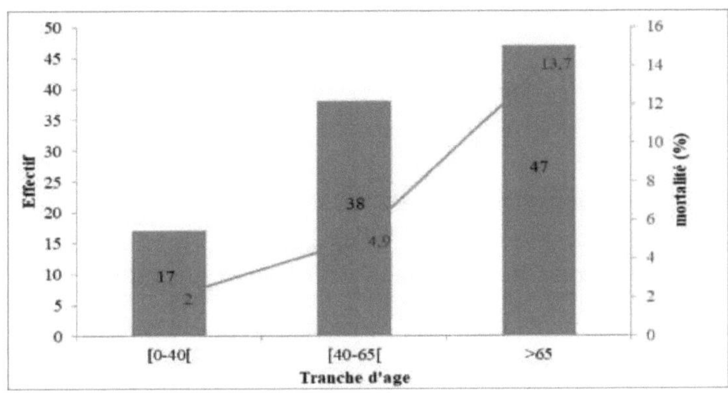

Figure 15 Mortality by age group

Table III: Cross-tabulation of deaths and age group

Age group (years)	Deaths		Total
	N	%	
0-40	2	2	17
41-65	5	4,9	38
>65	14	13,7	47
total	21	20,6	**102**

1.4.1.2.2 Gender

The breakdown of deaths by sex showed a predominance of males. Fifteen male deaths (25.9%) were reported, compared with 6 female deaths (13.6%), with a statistically insignificant difference (p=0.13).

Table IV: Breakdown of deaths by gender

Décès	**Sexe**		**Total**
	Femme	Homme	
Non	38	43	81
Oui	6	15	21
%	13,6	25,9	-
Total	44	58	102

1.4.1.2.3 Socio-economic level

In our population, most of the patients who died (n=21) had a good to average socioeconomic level, with a statistically significant association (p=0.01).

1.4.1.2.4 Comorbidities

We looked possible correlations between mortality and the number of comorbidities, the Charlson score and the type of comorbidity. A statistically

significant relationship was found between mortality and the Charlson score (p=0.004).
Patients with a history of diabetes, hypertension or ischaemic heart disease were statistically more exposed to the risk of death (Table V).

Mortality was high in patients with a BMI of less than 18, reaching 47.1%, with a statistically significant association (p=0.001) (Table VI).

Table V: Breakdown of deaths by comorbidity

	Number of patients	Deaths N	Deaths %	p-value
				0.034
Diabetes	18	7	38,8	
HTA	28		1242,9	0,001
Ischaemic heart disease	10	5	50	0,015
COPD	21	7	33,3	0,1
Asthma	22	2	9,1	0,13
Reflux	32	4	12,5	0,17
Obesity	5	0	0	0,24
Measles	0	0	0	-

Table VI: Breakdown of deaths by weight status

Deaths	**Weight status**										**Total**
	<18		18-24		25-29		30-40		>40		-
	n	%	n	%	n	%	n	%	n	%	
No	9	52,9	26	68,4	38	97,4	7	100	1	100	81
Yes	8	47,1	12	31,6	1	2,6	0	0	0	0	21
Total	**17**		**38**		**39**		**7**		**1**		**102**

1.4.1.2.5 Quality of life

The St Georges questionnaire could not be administered to patients who had died, which prevented us from estimating quality of life in this particular case.

1.4.1.2.6 Cigarette smoking

Twelve deaths involved active cigarette smokers. The average number of packs per year was 26. The association was not statistically significant (p=0.25).

1.4.1.2.7 Haemoptysis

Five deaths occurred among patients with haemoptysis. The association was not statistically significant (p= 0.51). The abundance of haemoptysis was low in patients who died (p= 0.28). Recurrence of haemoptysis in these patients was observed in 2 cases (p=0.21).

1.4.1.2.8 Number of exacerbations

The average number of exacerbations was 2 with extremes of 1 to 12 exacerbations/year. There was a peak in deaths at 9 for patients with 2 exacerbations per year. The association was statistically significant (p=0.034) (Figure 16).

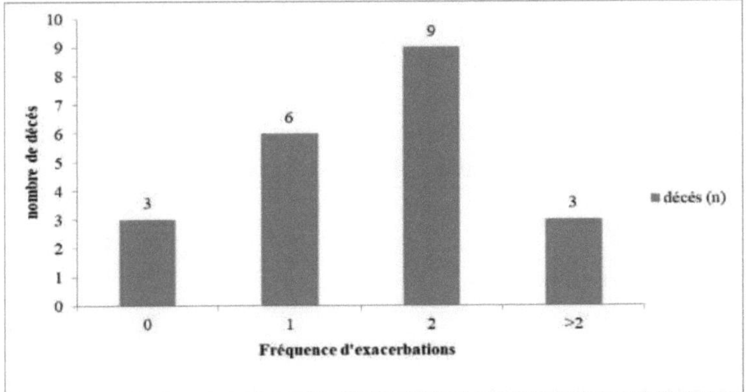

Figure 16: Breakdown of deaths by frequency of exacerbations

1.4.1.2.9 Number of hospitalisations

The average number of hospitalisations was 1.42 over the previous 2 years. We observed a peak in morality coinciding with patients having a history of hospitalisation in the previous 2 years. The association was statistically significant (p=0.004). No deaths were noted in patients who had not been hospitalised in the previous two years.

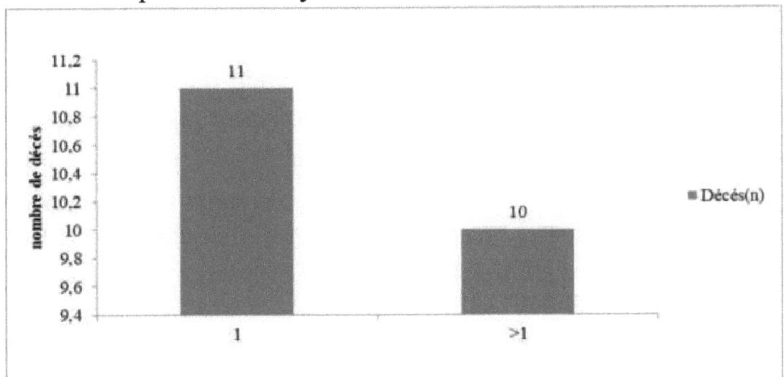

Figure 17 : Breakdown of deaths by frequency of hospitalisation

1.4.1.2.10 Infection

The presence of a history of superinfection by Pseudomonas was observed in 19 patients, 2 of whom died. No correlation was established with mortality in our

population. (p=0.49)
Pseudomonas colonisation occurred in 4 patients, only 1 of whom died. No correlation was established with mortality. (p=0,82)
We looked for possible superinfection by germs other than Pseudomonas. Similarly, no statistical association was found with mortality. We have illustrated the results for the various germs in the attached table. Colonisation by one of these germs was not found in our series in order to study its relationship with mortality.

Table VIICorrelation between death and the various microorganisms detected by the ECBC

Germ	n	Deaths		P
		n	%	
Pseudomonas Aeruginosa	19	2	11	0,49
Aspergillosis	3	0	0	0,57
Branhamella catarrhalis	5	2	40	0,27
Candida albicans	2	0	0	0,46
E.Coli	1	0	0	0,60
Haemophilus Influenzae	4	1	25	0,82
Pneumococcus	3	1	33	0,57
Kleibsielle pneumoniae	1	0	0	0,6
Acinetobacter Baumani	1	0	0	0,60
Serratia Marcosuras	2	1	50	0,29

1.4.1.2.11 Respiratory function

We looked for a possible relationship between the percentage of FEV1 in the 4 groups and survival in our population. We obtained the following results: no deaths were found in the mild group, unlike the other groups, in which 6, 10 and 5 deaths were found respectively in the moderate, severe and very severe groups (p=0.034).
An analysis mortality using Kaplan and Meier survival showed no statistically significant difference between the 4 groups (p=0.71).

1.4.1.2.12 Type DDB

We studied the relationship between the 3 types of DDB and mortality (bearing in mind that they may be associated). The number of deaths was not significantly different according to the type of DDB and also according to the presence or absence of emphysema and hilar or mediastinal adenopathies. The number of deaths was 20%, 19% and 19% respectively for cylindrical, cystic and moniliform types (table VIII).

Table VIII: Distribution of deaths according to radiological abnormalities radiological abnormalities on chest CT

Type	n	Deaths		P
		n	%	
Cylindrical	75		1520	0,86
Moniliform	37	7	19	0,89
Cystic	59		1119	0,77
Associations	53	9	17	0,48
Emphysema	31	8	26	0,38
Adenopathies mediastinal/hilar	35	7	20	0,91

1.4.1.2.13 Etiology

The aetiologies found were characterised by their variability. Pulmonary tuberculosis was diagnosed in 19 patients, 4 of whom died (21.1%). DDB secondary to severe infectious pneumopathy during childhood was found in 9 patients, only 1 of whom died. Similarly, a systemic disease was diagnosed in 7 patients, 2 of whom died, and a single case of vasculitis (Wegener's) with no known cause of death.

No statistical relationship was established between the various aetiologies and mortality (Table IX).

Table IX: Breakdown of deaths by etiology of DDB

Etiology	N	Deaths		P
		n	%	
Tuberculosis	19		421,1	0,95
Post-infectious	9		111,1	0,46
Systemic disease	7		228,6	0,58
Idiopathic	67		1420,9	0,91
Total	102		2120,6	

1.4.1.2.14 Treatment

We found no relationship between mortality and treatment, except for the use of Bromhexine (p=0.034).

Table X: Mortality as a function of treatment

Medicines	N	Deaths		P
		n	%	
Inhaled corticosteroids	64	13	61,9	0,93
LAMA	8	2	9,5	0,75

LABA	40	8	38,1	0,91
Theophyline	21	4	19	0,85
Bromhexine	40	4	19	0,034
Surgery	8	2	25	0,75
OLD and/or NIV	25	7	28	0,24
Respiratory physiotherapy	14	2	14	0,53

1.4.2 Severity scores

BSI and FACED scores

We studied the variables defining the FACED and BSI scores. The distribution of patients by variable according to each score is shown in Tables 9 and 10.

We then studied the characteristics of patients in each of the 3 risk groups for each score and found a difference in the distribution of patients according to the score used.

1.4.2.1 FACED score

Using the FACED score, the results were as follows: the "mild" group comprised 32 patients (31.4%), the "moderate" group 48 patients (47%) and the "severe" group 22 patients (21.6%).

Table XI: The FACED score

Variable	Sample (n=102)	
	n	%
FEV1		
<50%	56	55
>50%	46	45
Age (year)		
>70	33	32
<70	69	68
Colonisation by Pseudomonas Aeruginosa		
no	98	96
yes	4	4
Radiological extension		
>2 lobes	102	100
<2 lobes	0	0
Dyspnoea- mMRC		
> II (III and IV)	47	46
< II (0- II)	55	54

1.4.2.2 BSI score

The BSI score was used to classify patients into a "mild" group comprising 22 patients (21.6%), a "moderate" group comprising 21 patients (20.6%) and a "severe" group comprising 59 patients (57.8%).

Table XII: The BSI score

Variable	Sample (n=102)	
	N	%
Age (years) <50	46	45
50-69	31	30
70-79	14	14
>80	11	11
Body Mass Index (BMI) <18.5	9	9
>18.5	93	91
FEV1(%)		
>80%	12	12
50-80%	45	44
30-49%	31	30
<30%	14	14
Hospitalisations in the previous 2 years no	31	30
yes	71	70
Exacerbations in the previous year 0-2	72	71
>3	30	29
Dyspnoea - MRC 1-3	74	73
4	26	25
5	2	2
Colonisation by Pseudomonas Aeruginosa no	98	96
yes	4	4
Colonisation by another non	102	100
yes	0	0
Radiological extension (> 3 lobes and/or cystic DDB)		
no	61	59
yes	41	41

1.4.2.3 Link between BSI and FACED scores

A bi-variate study showed a statistically significant relationship between BSI and FACED scores (Pearson test, p<0.0001).

Table XIII: Classification of patients by FACED and BSI scores

BSI	FACED			
	Light	**moderate**	**Severe**	**Total**
Light	14 (43,8%)	5 (104%)	3 (13,6%)	22 (21,6%)
Moderate	6 (18,8%)	14 (29,2%)	1 (4,5%)	21 (20,6%)
Severe	12 (37,5%)	29 (60,4%)	18 (81,8%)	59 (57,8%)
Total	32 (31,4%)	48 (47,1%)	22 (21,6%)	102 (100%)

1.4.2.4 Severity scores and mortality

The BSI score was more sensitive than the FACED score in predicting mortality with a greater area under the curve (AUC) (0.77 versus 0.67) and a lower more significant p-value (p<0.0001).

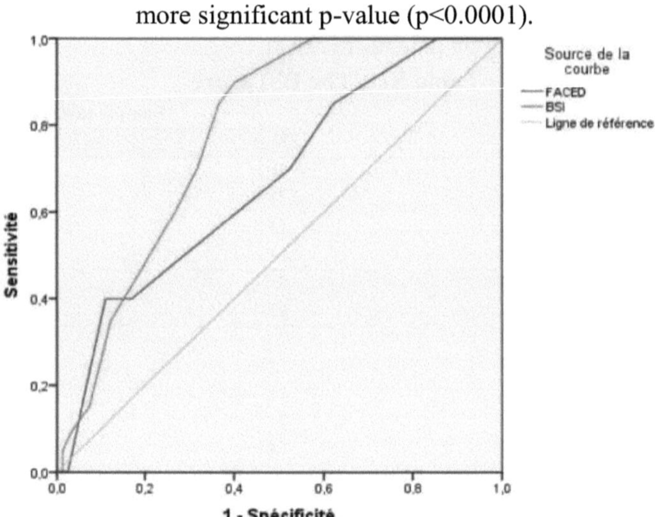

Figure 18: ROC curve: Mortality according to FACED and BSI scores

1.4.2.5 Severity scores and prediction of hospital admissions

Patients hospitalised once during the previous two years were mainly in the severe and moderate groups for the BSI and FACED score respectively, with superiority for the BSI since it includes 24 patients compared with 18 for FACED. If we look at patients hospitalised more than once in the previous two years, we find 34 patients classified as severe BSI versus 18 moderate FACED patients. (table XIV)

The BSI score was more sensitive than the FACED score in predicting hospitalisations, with a higher AUC (0.95 versus 0.69) and a more significant p-value (p<0.0001).

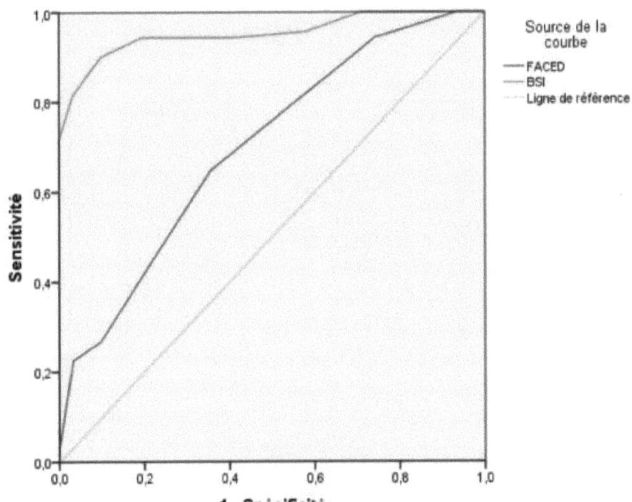

Figure 19: ROC curve: Hospitalisations according to FACED and BSI scores

Table XIV: Breakdown of hospital admissions by severity score severity score

	Hospitalization n=1			Hospitalization n >1		
	Light	Moderate	Severe	Light	Moderate	Severe
BSI	4	7	24	0	2	34
FACED	10	18	7	6	18	12

1.4.2.6 Severity scores and prediction of exacerbations

Patients who had had 2 exacerbations in the previous year were mainly in the severe and moderate groups for the BSI and FACED scores respectively (11 patients versus 13 respectively). More frequent exacerbations in excess of 2 were observed in patients classified as severe by the BSI score (28) and in the moderate group by the FACED score (15). (Table XV).

The difference between the two scores was not significant, with AUCs of 0.65 and 0.64 respectively for the FACED and BSI scores and a similar p-value (p=0.02). These results show that the 2 scores are not very sensitive in predicting exacerbations since their corresponding AUCs do not exceed 0.7.

Table XV: Distribution of exacerbations according to severity score severity score

	Exacerbation n=2			Exacerbation n >2		
	Light	Moderate	Severe	Light	Moderate	Severe[1]
BSI	4	6	11	1	1	28

FACED	5	13	3	8	15	7

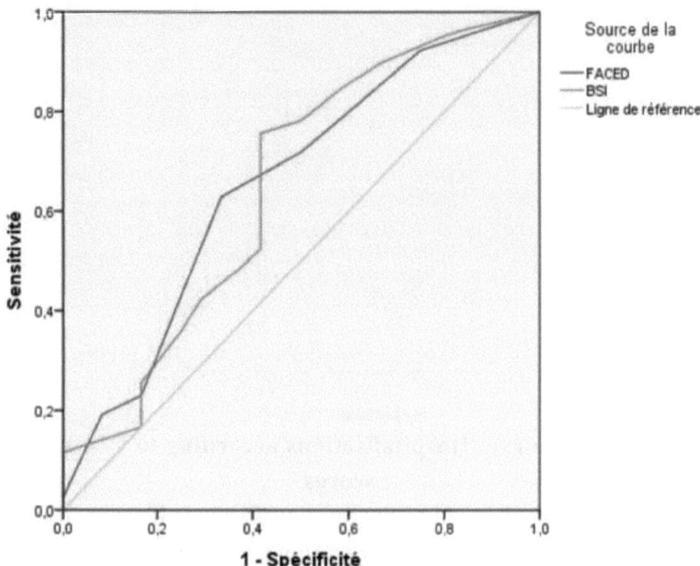

Figure 20: ROC curve: exacerbations according to FACED and BSI

1.4.2.7 Severity scores and survival

The distribution of deaths within the risk groups showed their predominance in the severe group for the BSI, where the majority of patients died (20 patients) with only one patient belonging to the moderate group, unlike the FACED score, where the distribution of deaths was as follows: 3 in the mild group (10%), 10 in the moderate group (21%) and 8 in the severe group (36%). (Table XVI)

Table XVI: Number of deaths according to severity score

	Subjects	Deaths
	N	N%
BSI		
Light	22	00
Moderate	21	15
Severe	59	2034
FACED		
Light	32	310
Moderate	48	1021
Severe	22	836

We constructed the Kaplein and Meyer ten-year survival curves according to FACED and BSI scores. curves differed according to the severity score used.
For the BSI score: The survival curve showed significant early mortality in the severe group. Mortality in the mild and moderate groups was not significant, and the survival curve in this case was horizontal.
For the FACED score: mortality is highest in the moderate and severe groups, with a rapidly declining survival curve, particularly for the severe group.

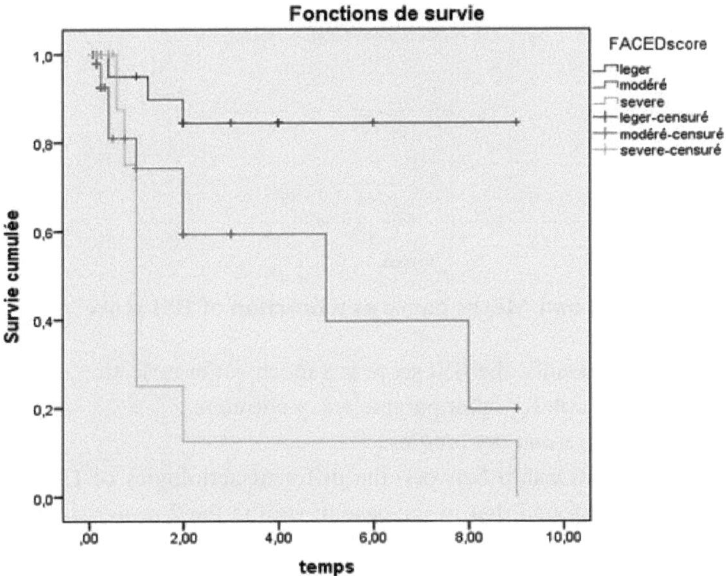

Figure 21: Kaplein and Meyer curve as a function of FACED score

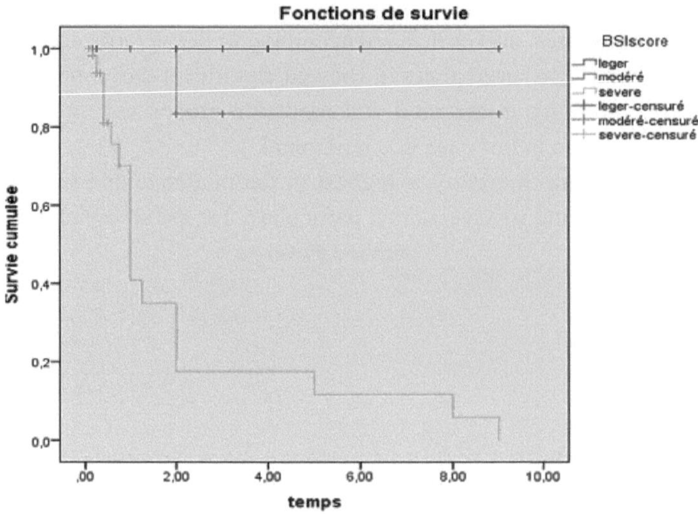

Figure 22: Kaplein and Meyer curve as a function of BSI score

According to these results, the BSI score is a much better reflection of reality. To do this, we will look for other parameters y correlate.

1.4.2.8 Severity scores and aetiologies

We studied the relationship between the different aetiologies of DDB and the severity scores, and found that in the case of COPD the 2 scores diverged. The BSI score classifies the majority of COPD patients (81%) in the severe group, with a statistically significant relationship (Figure 23). This is not the case for the FACED score, where only 21% are severe (Figure 24). No difference was found for the other aetiologies.

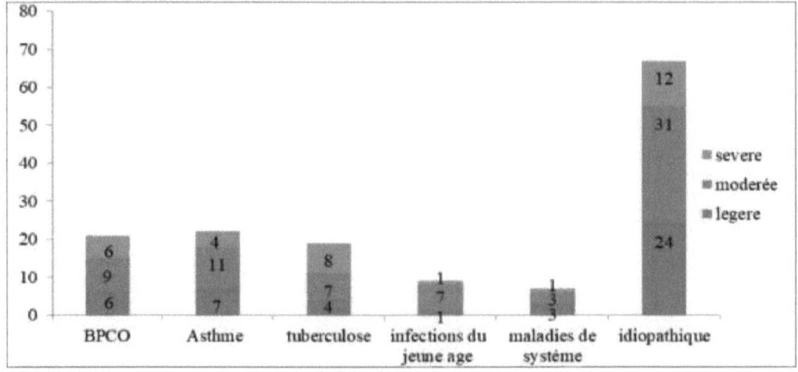

Figure 23: Distribution of etiologies of DDB according to FACED

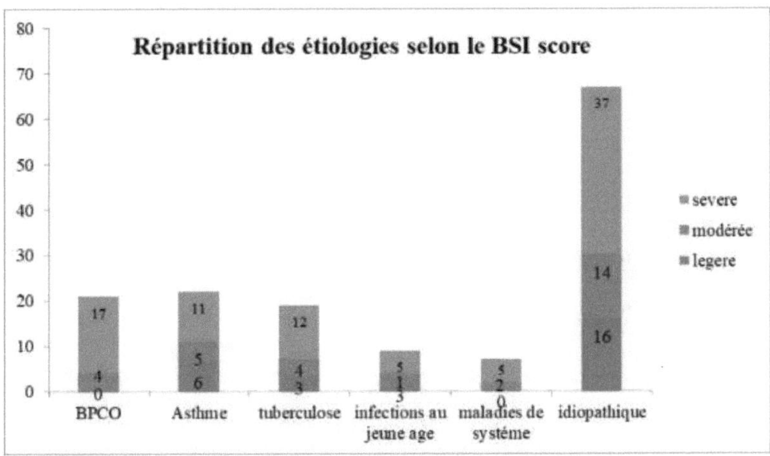

Figure 24: Distribution of aetiologies according to BSI score

1.4.2.9 Severity scores and radiological damage :

We looked for a possible relationship between the type of bronchiectasis, the number of lobes affected, hilar and mediastinal adenopathies and emphysema with the FACED and BSI scores. Our results were in favour of a statistically significant relationship between an association of 2 or more of the types of DDB with the 2 scores. However, this relationship differed according to the score used.

In fact, if we used the FACED, we would have 30 patients classified as moderate in severity, whereas the BSI classifies more patients (37 cases) as severe (Figures 25 and 26). The BSI score is therefore a better reflection of radiological severity.

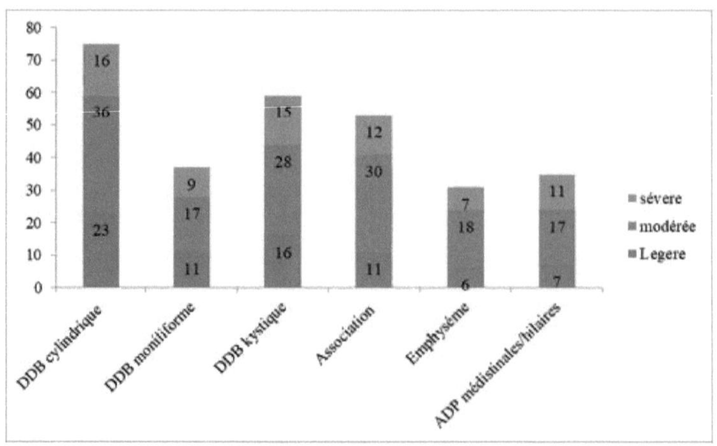

Figure 25: Distribution of radiological lesions according to FACED score

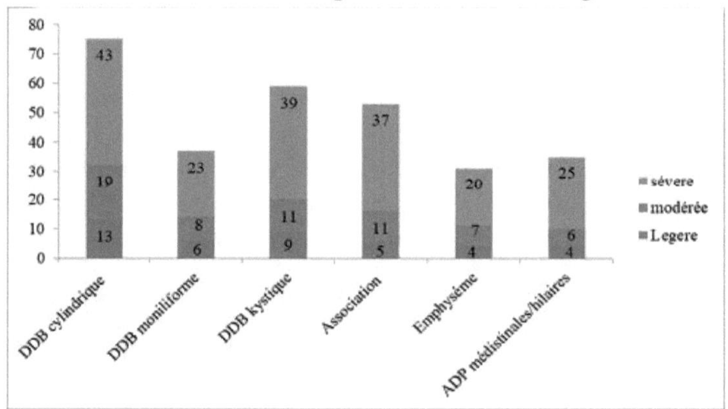

Figure 26: Distribution of radiological lesions according to BSI score

1.4.2.10 Severity scores and FEV1

There was a significant statistical relationship between the FEV1 value and the two severity scores ($p<0.001$).

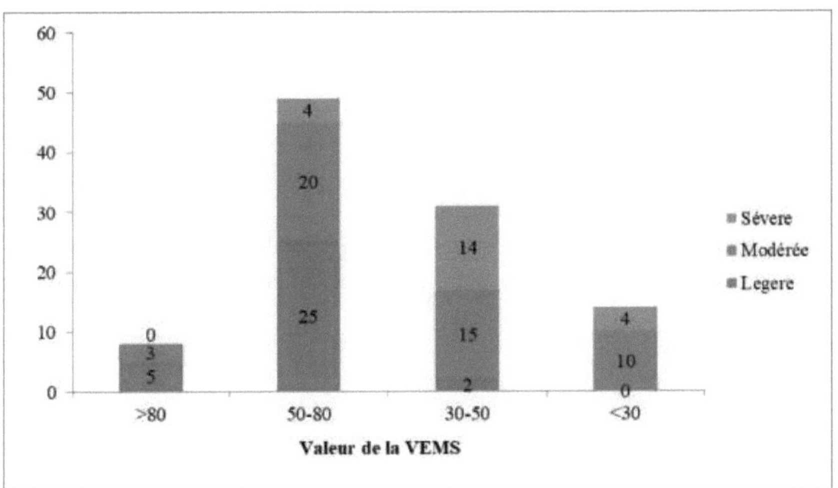

Figure 27: Distribution of patients according to FACED score and FEV1

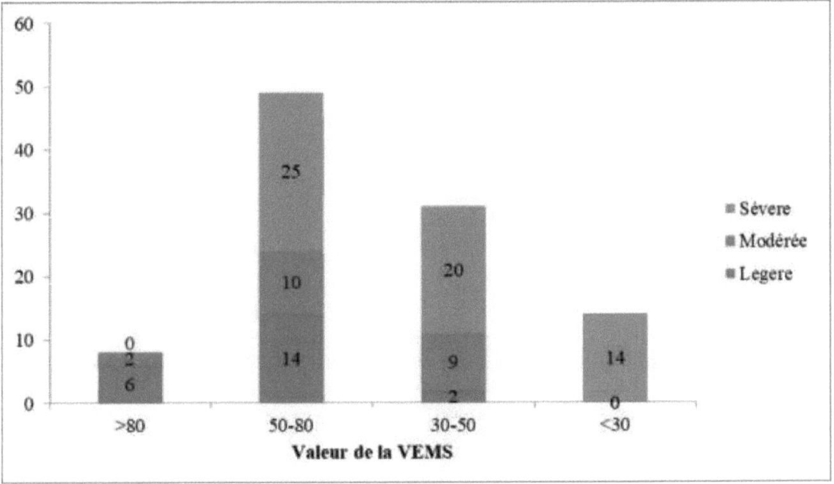

Figure 28: Distribution of patients according to BSI score and FEV1

1 .4.2.11 Severity scores and Quality of Life

Quality of life was estimated on the basis of the SGRQ. We calculated the 3 components of the score: symptoms, activity and impact in order obtain the total SGRQ. To do this, we excluded from our population deceased patients for whom the questionnaire had not been completed. This gave us 82 patients.

The median of the total SGRQ varied according to the severity score used. Looking at the BSI score, median total SGRQ was equal to 67 and corresponded to the severe group. The other moderate and mild groups had a total SGRQ of 50 and 47 respectively. For the FACED score, the median SGRQ was virtually the same in the moderate and severe groups, with values of 65 and 64

respectively, and lower at around 44 in the mild group (Figures 29 and 30).
We did not find a statistically significant relationship between the SGRQ and the severity scores, the p-values were equal to 0.7 and 0.44 respectively for the BSI and FACED scores (Fisher's exact test). Similarly, no statistical relationship was found between the 3 parts of the SGRQ (symptom, activity and impact) with the BSI and FACED scores (Table XVII).
On the other hand, there was a significant statistical relationship between the SGRQ and the HAD scale, the number of exacerbations and hospitalisations (Table XVIII).

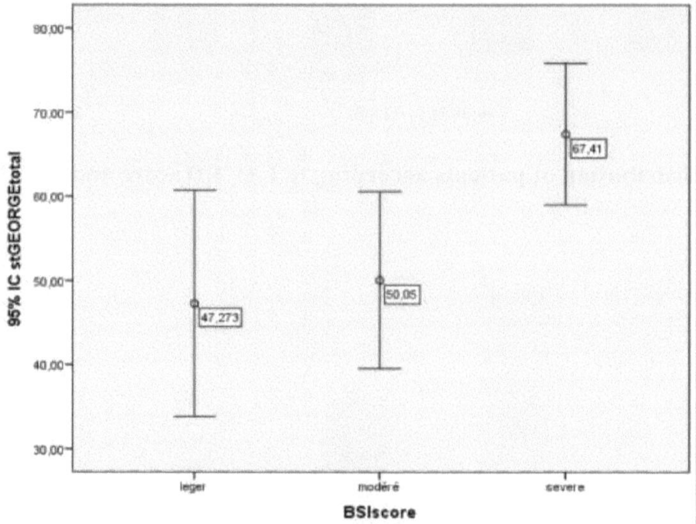

Figure 29Total SGRQ in each severity group according to BSI score

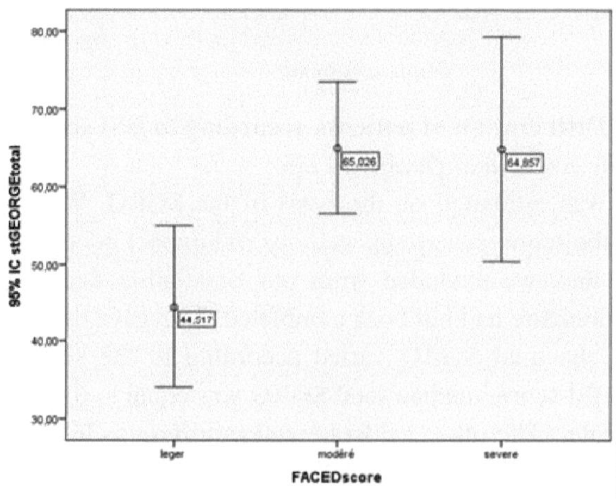

Figure 30: Total SGRQ in each severity group according to FACED score

Table XVII: Distribution of patients according to SGRQ and severity scores

severity scores

Severity score		SGRQ symptoms	SGRQ activity	SGRQ total	SGRQ impact
FACED	Light 42	48	41	44	
	Moderate	65	64	65	65
	Severe	65	63	63	64
BSI	Light 46	51	45	47	
	Moderate	52	47	46	50
	Severe	65	68	68	67

Table XVIII: Estimation of quality of life according to the SGRQ as a function of

severity scores

	Scale HAH	Number exacerbations/year	Number hospital admissions/year	OLD/VNI
SGRQ total	<0,001	<0.001	0,006	0,001

1.4.2.12 Severity scores and psychological status :

In order to assess the psychological status of our patients, we used the HAD scale, which assesses anxiety and depression. A total score (anxiety+depression) greater than 15 or a component (anxiety or depression) greater than 11 indicates the presence of an anxiety or depressive disorder in the patient. We identified 45 patients with an anxiety-depression disorder among 81 patients, i.e. 55.6%.

The distribution of these patients differed according to the severity score used. Using the FACED score, 27 patients (60%) were classified as moderate, whereas using the BSI score, 27 patients were classified as severe. On the other hand, using the BSI score, 27 patients would be classified in the severe group (Table XIX).

The statistical relationship between the HAD scale and the 2 severity scores was significant, ***with*** p-values of around 0.004 and 0.039 for the FACED and BSI scores respectively.

Table XIX: Estimate of psychological status using the HAD scale as a function of

according to severity scores

Severity score	Positive HAD scale

	Light	9
FACED	Moderate	27
	Severe	9
	Light	8
BSI	Moderate	10
	Severe	27

1.4.3 Multivariate study of mortality

Binary logistic regression was used to search for independent risk factors for mortality in our population. We found 8 factors: number of co-morbidities, GERD, associated asthma, hypertension, medium to high socio-economic level, number of hospitalisations/2 years, isolation of Branhamella catarrhalis, non-use of Bromhexin.

Table XX: Risk factors for mortality after multivariate study

Variables	A	RR (95% CI)	p-value
Gender	-1,61	0,58	0,45
Age	-0,054	0,28	0,59
High socio-economic level	3,58	36,37	0.006
Average socio-economic level	2,77	13,33	0,038
BMI	-0,67	0,000	0,62
HTA	2,6	3,6	0.3
Diabetes	-0,2	0,00	0,996
COPD	-1,58	0,13	0,71
Asthma	-4,011	3,032	0,082
Ischaemic heart disease	-1,05	0,01	0,998
GERD	-4,71	0.012	0.005
Number of co-morbidities	1,14	6,13	0.001
CCI	0,44	0,29	0,59
Abundance of haemoptysis	12-13	1,14	0,77
Recurrence of haemoptysis	0,14	1,5	0,88
Branhamella Catarrhalis	1,44	1,39	0,24
Hospital admissions/2 years	-1,72	1,33	0,25
Interval between hospitalisations	4,75	3,15	0,043
Exacerbations/1 year	-0,46	0,13	0,71
Bromhexine (not used)	1,06	2,89	0,27

CHAPTER III

Results

1. Epidemiology

1.1 Incidence

Depending on the country

DDB is a major public health problem in Tunisia and throughout the world, and is responsible for considerable healthcare costs. For a long time, this condition was under-diagnosed, until the advent of the multi-band thoracic scanner, which played a major role in its diagnosis.

In Europe, the number of hospital admissions for DDB is rising sharply, with an average of 2.9% per year in Germany between 2005 and 2011 (18). In Spain, it is estimated that the prevalence of DDB varies between 42 and 566/100,000 inhabitants(14).

In the UK, the prevalence of DDB in women increased from 350.5 per 100,000 population in 2004 to 566.1 per 100,000 population in 2013, and in men from 301.2 per 100,000 population in 2004 to 485.5 per 100,000 population in 2013 (2).

In the United States, Seitz et al (2012) reported an increase in annual prevalence to 8.7% (19).

In South Korea (20), the incidence of DDB is estimated at 464/100,000 inhabitants. It is therefore considered that DDB is not uncommon, especially as the annual cost of care for these patients is EUR 218.

In Tunisia, despite recent studies on this pathology, none of them has estimated the real prevalence of DDB. What is known is that it is a frequent cause of hospitalisation in pneumology.

Our study involved 110 cases of diffuse DDB followed up in the Pneumology Department of the Hédi Chaker Hospital in Sfax.

By gender

Male involvement was predominant in our study, contrary to what is reported in the literature. In Europe, a meta-analysis (10) of 7 European cohorts (Scotland, Ireland, Italy, Belgium, Greece, England, Serbia) showed a predominance of females in all cohorts. Similarly, in the United States (USA), the American Bronchial Dilatation Research Registry (21) counted 1,826 cases of bronchial dilatation collected between 2008 and 2014, 76% of whom were female. A selection bias may explain this difference, as we were particularly interested in diffuse DDB, which may influence the results.

Table XXI: Breakdown of series by gender

	Study period	Men(%)	Female(%)
Our study	2009-2019	58	42
Scotland	2011-2015	39,3	60,7
Ireland	2008-2015	32 ,9	67,1
Italy	2011-2015	41,2	58,8
Belgium	2006-2012	49	51
Greece	2010-2015	36	64
Angletaire	2009-2013	40,5	59,5
Serbia	2010-2015	29,2	70,8
USA	2008-2014	24	76

According to age

The immune system is less effective in young children and the elderly, leading to an increased incidence of infection in these two groups(22). DDB has most often been described as beginning in childhood, particularly in the first five years of life, with a tendency to improve significantly in late adolescence and then a worsening of symptoms by the age of 50 to 60(23,24). Nowadays, this condition is described more frequently in the elderly (22).

In Europe, the average age of patients with DDB varies between 59 and 66, according to a meta-analysis of 7 European cohorts (10).

In the United States, the American Registry of Bronchial Dilatation Research showed an average age of 64±14 years. The predominant age group was between 50 and 79 years (21).

In our study, the average age was 60, with extremes ranging from 16 to 90, and a peak in the over-70s.

Table XXII: Average age of patients by series

series	Study period	Average age
Our study	2009-2019	60
Scotland	2011-2015	65,3
Ireland	2008-2015	60,5
Italy	2011-2015	65,1
Belgium	2006-2012	66,4
Greece	2010-2015	59,3
England	2009-2013	59,1
Serbia	2010-2015	62
USA	2008-2014	64

1.2 Clinical study

1.2.1 Habits (smoking)

Active and passive exposure to tobacco smoke is well known as a major risk factor for chronic respiratory disease.

In Europe, a meta-analysis involved 7 prospective European cohorts: Monza, Italy; Dundee and New Castle, United Kingdom; Louvain, Belgium; Barcelona, Spain; Athens, Greece; Galway, Ireland. It studied 1258 cases of DDB, 36% of whom had a history of smoking (25).

In Turkey, a prospective study was carried out by Onen et al on 98 cases of DDB (12) . It showed that 24.5% of patients were smokers, with a mean of 8.69±18.11 PA.

In the United States, the percentage of smokers has been estimated at 40% (21).

In our study, smoking was more frequent than in the literature, at 45% with an average of 26 PA. This may be explained by the increasingly high smoking rate. Only 24 people were weaned off smoking.

1.2.2 Personal history

In the UK, Jennifer et al studied 18793 cases of DDB between 2004 and 2013. She showed that 63.4% of patients with DDB had at least one concomitant disease. Asthma was the most common condition (42.5%), followed by COPD (36.1%) (2).

In Turkey, 53% of patients had at least one comorbidity, including cardiovascular disease (19.4%), hypertension (21.4%) and diabetes (5.1%).

In Europe, Sara et al found that COPD associated with DDB occurred in 15% of cases, whereas asthma was less frequent (3, 25).

In our study, a personal medical history was common, accounting for 84% of cases. GERD was the most common (29%). Other antecedents were reported notably hypertension (27%), asthma (20%), COPD (19%), diabetes (17%) and finally cardiovascular antecedents (coronary artery disease and rhythm or conduction disorders) in 15% of cases.

In fact, gastro resophageal reflux disease (GERD) is not uncommon in chronic respiratory diseases. In Australia, the prevalence of both symptomatic and non-symptomatic GERD has been estimated by Lee et al to be between 26 and 75%, with a significant incidence of micro aspiration of gastric fluid into the tracheobronchial tree (26).

Based on the various comorbidities, the Charlson score was established. Thirteen patients had a negative CCI, with the majority of patients having a score between 1 and 4 (66%).

1.2.3 Reason for consultation

In the United States, the American registry of research on DDB (21) described the main symptoms reported by patients: cough (73%), which is productive in 53% of cases, dyspnoea (64%) and fatigue (50%).

In Europe, a meta-analysis showed that 75% of patients had a chronic cough,

62% a morning bronchorrhoea and 15% haemoptysis (25).
These results differ from our own because of the variability of symptoms during the course of DDB. In our population, exertional dyspnoea was predominant (99%). Chronic productive cough was also frequent (82%), as were morning bronchorrhoea (46%), chest pain (31%), lower respiratory infections (26%) and haemoptysis (25%). This difference may be explained by epidemiological and aetiological changes depending on geographical origin of patients around the world (27).

1.3 Paraclinical study

1.3.1 Thoracic imaging: Contribution of multi-bar thoracic CT scans

Multi-band chest CT is currently the GOLD standard for diagnosing DDB. It also plays an important role in determining the severity of the disease, as it forms part of the FACED and BSI scores.

1.3.1.1 Number of lobes affected

In our study, we were particularly interested in diffuse DDB, primarily for epidemiological reasons, since this is the most common type of DDB in the world and in our country. Indeed, in a multicentre study, Lynch et al found that localised DDB represented only 5% of the population (28). The results were no different in the United States, where only 11% of patients had localised DDB (21). Similarly, a Spanish meta-analysis (8) showed an average of 2.52±1.2 lobes affected.
Secondly, our interest in DDB, particularly diffuse DDB, is justified since it appears to be more severe according to the literature (23).

1.3.1.2 Types of DDB

However, identification of the three types of DDB (cylindrical, moniliform, cystic) is of little clinical interest and does not help to orientate the aetiological work-up. On the other hand, cystic bronchiectasis is associated with a poorer prognosis in terms of functional decline, sputum purulence and growth of Pseudomonas Aeruginosa (28).
In our study, cylindrical DDB predominated (75%), followed by cystic forms (56%). Loubeyre et al (29) demonstrated in a retrospective study carried out in France that 45% of patients had emphysema associated with lesions of DDB, highlighting the relationship between emphysema and the radiological extension and severity of DDB. In our study, emphysema was frequent, affecting 30.4% of patients. This may be due, on the one hand, to the radiological extension since we interested in diffuse DDB and, on the other hand, to the non-negligible prevalence of associated COPD (15%).

1.3.2 Sputum cytobacteriological examination (SCC)

Respiratory infection represents an evolutionary turning point in the course of

DDB, hence the interest in identifying microorganisms in the patient's sputum, both during exacerbations and in the stable state, in order to look for probable colonisation (30).
Pseudomonas Aeruginosa and Haemophilus influenzae (HI) are the two most frequently isolated bacteria worldwide, although the proportions vary between countries and populations (27). A meta-analysis by Finchk et al (31) in 2015 of 3,683 patients with DDB showed that 21.4% of patients were colonised by pyocyanins and that mortality, frequency of hospitalisation and exacerbations were three times higher in these patients than in non-colonised subjects. More recently, in 2019, a prospective study was conducted by Amorim et al (30), which showed that colonisation by HI and Pseudomonas Aeruginosa was frequent in Portugal, reaching 32.3% and 30.1% respectively.
Our results differ from those reported in the literature. In fact, colonisation by Pseudomonas Aeruginosa was identified in only 4 patients (3.6%). On the other hand, a history of superinfection by the same germ without being able to meet the definition of colonisation represented 17.3% of our population. These results may be explained by the fact that in the majority of cases, and particularly in stable patients, it is not common practice to request an ECBC.

1.3.3 Functional respiratory investigation

It should be carried out in a stable state, outside infectious flare-ups. Patients with bronchiectasis have no particular functional profile. The abnormalities observed reflect the extent of the lesions, their severity and any associated respiratory diseases.
According to the 2018 Spanish recommendations (14), an obstructive syndrome is observed in most patients, particularly in subjects who smoke and/or have COPD. The association with a restrictive syndrome is frequent, generally due to the presence of atelectatic or non-ventilated territories due to obstructive secretions, this can be seen during pulmonary tuberculosis and in destructive fibrosing forms.
Measurement of FEV1 is essential for calculating severity scores. A meta-analysis (25) showed a median FEV1 of 73%. A prospective study in Brazil (32) showed a mean FEV1 value of 48±14.8%.
In Tunisia, we have no other studies evaluating the functional profile of patients with DDB. Our results do not differ from those in the literature, since obstructive ventilatory disorders predominate in 44.5% of cases, and restrictive disorders to a lesser extent in 27.3%. The mean FEV1 value in our population was 52%.

2. Mortality

To date, we not have enough studies on mortality during DDB. This condition,

which used to be considered harmless, is no longer so, since recent studies have shown its impact on patient survival and quality of life.
Loebinger et al (5) were able to follow patients with DDB over a period of 14 years in a study validating the SGRQ in DDB. The authors were able to describe in detail the impact of DDB on mortality: 29.7% of patients died during follow-up, a figure that was double that expected on the basis of life expectancy for individuals in the United Kingdom. The cause of death was respiratory in 70.4% of cases.
Other studies have shown significant mortality associated with DDB, notably in Turkey (16.3%) with an estimated mean survival of 44.06±1.6 months (12). In Belgium (33), a study showed a prevalence of DDB of 539 cases among 20998 patients consulting for respiratory disease, i.e. 2.6%. Mortality was high at 10.6%.
In Germany, on the other hand, mortality remained stable between 2005 and 2011, estimated at 0.003/100,000 inhabitants, which is a low value (18).
In South Korea, it is estimated that 2.9% of patients with DDB die in hospital, and that 1.4% die specifically from DDB (20).
In Tunisia, we did not find any studies that could used to assess the mortality associated with DDB. Our results are similar to those in the literature, with a high mortality rate of around 19.1%. The risk factors for mortality were studied and will be detailed later.

Table XXIII: Mortality by series

series	Kingdom Uni	Turkey	Belgium	South Korea south	Our study
Study period	1994	2000-2005	2006-2009	2012-2017	2018-2019
Number of cases	111	98	539	1, 400,000	110
Mortality (%)	29,7	16,3	10,6	2,9	19.1

3. Prognostic factors

Several factors can influence the severity of DDB. These include epidemiological factors such as age, gender, co-morbidities, clinical factors, lung function, radiological abnormalities, genetics, microbiology and systemic inflammation. All these factors have been well studied in a review of the literature (34) and are summarised in table XXIV.

Table XXIV: Factors influencing the prognosis of DDB in the literature

Clinical parameters	Good prognosis or mild DDB	Poor prognosis or severe DDB
Bacteriology	No germs	**Pseudomonas Aeruginosa**

	No colonisation by HI	Staphylococci Aureus Methy R Gram-negative Enterobacteriaceae High bacterial load
Radiology	< 3 lobes Cylindrical DDBs	**> 3 lobes** **Cystic DDB** **Thickening of the bronchial wall** **Mosaic infusion** **Emphysema** Mucous plugs
Function Respiratory	EFR normal	**Obstructive ventilatory disorder** Restrictive ventilatory disorder High VR/CPT Low DLCO
Dyspnoea on exertion	No exertional dyspnoea	**Dyspnoea stage 4/5 MRC**
Symptoms	Sputum volume < 5 ml/d Mucous or mucopurulent phlegm Occasional coughing or coughing up during exacerbations	Sputum volume >25 ml/d **Stable purulent sputum** Persistent cough
Etiology	No co-morbidities	**Associated COPD** Associated PR
Exacerbations	<3/year	>3/year **Severe exacerbations requiring hospitalisation**

3.1 Epidemiological data

3.1.1 Age and gender

Loebinger et al (5) studied the mortality risk factors associated with DDB over a period of 13 years. They found that 29.7% of patients died, whereas the normal percentage of deaths estimated by the national statistics office is 14.7% in men and 8.9% in women of the same age. The average age of patients who died of DDB was 60. A multi-varied study concluded that age and male sex are independent risk factors for mortality.

In Germany, Felix et al (18) studied the frequency of hospitalisation related DDB. According to the authors, the highest value was 39.4 hospitalisations/100,000 inhabitants among men aged between 75 and 84. German statistics also showed that there were 164 reported deaths due to DDB, including 93 men and 71 women. Of the patients who died, 131 (80%) were aged >65 and 80 (49%) were aged >70.

Similarly, in Turkey, Onen et al (12) showed that the mean age of patients who died was significantly higher than that of survivors: 72 compared with 59.7 years. The results of the multi-varied study confirmed that age is an independent

risk factor for mortality, but this was not the case gender.
Our study is consistent with the literature, and the mean age was statistically higher in patients who died. Mortality increased with age, but after multivariate analysis, age was not an independent risk factor for mortality. The distribution of deaths by sex showed a non-significant predominance of males. The multivariate study concluded that gender was not a risk factor for mortality.

3.1.2 Co-morbidities

As with COPD, DDB may be associated with one or more co-morbidities that affect the prognosis of the disease. It is for this reason that teams have been interested in studying this relationship. Melissa et al (35) have shown that the number and nature of comorbidities are risk factors for mortality in patients followed for DDB. Mortality increased by 17% with each addition a comorbidity. A total of 81 comorbidities were identified, 13 of which were considered to be potentially associated with increased mortality and were subsequently included in a BACI (Bronchiectasis Aetiology Comorbidity Index) score. These comorbidities included those considered to be significantly associated with mortality, such as COPD, metastatic cancer, connective tissue diseases, asthma and chronic inflammatory diseases of the digestive tract. Men had significantly more comorbidities than women, with a median of 4 comorbidities.

COPD

The association between COPD and DDB has become a subject of current debate and has been identified as a particular phenotype associated with susceptibility to airway colonisation, increased respiratory symptoms with impaired quality of life and frequent exacerbations (36, 37).

Cardiovascular co-morbidities

In our population, co-morbidities tend to be cardiovascular, particularly diabetes, hypertension and ischaemic heart disease. The coexistence of cardiac pathologies makes it even more difficult to manage patients, particularly during periods of exacerbation when both pathologies may be involved. Furthermore, the combination of several cardiovascular risk factors, including diabetes, increases the risk of cardiac decompensation.

Gastro resophageal reflux disease

Gastro resophageal reflux disease (GERD) is common in our population and represents independent risk factor for mortality according to the multi-variate study. These results are consistent with the literature, as shown by Mandal et al (38), GERD is an independent factor in the risk of exacerbation and severity of DDB. In addition, a study by McDonnell et al (39) showed that GERD is present in 26-75% of cases in patients with BMD. These patients have more severe

DDB. However, the effect of treatment of GERD on the prognosis of BMD has not yet been established.
The Charlson score is considered to be one of the best known and most widely used comorbidity scores for chronic diseases, cited in over 9,500 publications. Seitz et al (19) clearly demonstrated in their 2010 prospective study that the Charlson score is a predictor of high healthcare costs in the United States. The authors pointed out that the CCI can be useful in identifying patients who will have a high cost of care.
Our results are consistent with those of the literature, with a statistically significant relationship between mortality and ICC in the bivariate study (p=0.004), but this relationship was not significant in the multivariate study (p=0.54).
It is also interesting to assess the number of comorbidities. In our study we found a significant statistical link with mortality after the multivariate study (p= 0.001). Thus the number of comorbidities is an independent risk factor for mortality, whatever the comorbidity.

3.2 Clinical features

DDB is a debilitating condition, with frequent clinical respiratory symptoms that may be resistant to pharmacological treatment. Several studies have sought to identify the respiratory symptoms associated with increased disease severity, while stressing the importance of assessing quality of life in these patients. Among the clinical signs, exertional dyspnoea and sputum volume have been described in several publications.
As shown by Martinez-García et al (6) in a prospective study 86 patients, exertional dyspnoea and sputum volume (in millilitres) are significantly correlated with SGRQ (multivariate study).
M.P Murray et al (40) studied the relationship between the colour of sputum and the severity of the disease. According to the authors, bacterial colonisation occurs in 5% of mucous sputum, 43.5% of mucopurulent sputum and 86.4% of purulent sputum in a stable state. After multivariate analysis, they were able to demonstrate that purulent sputum was associated with several independent factors, including bacterial colonisation, cystic DDB, FEV1 <80% and an age of onset of the disease before 45.
Our study did not reveal any relationship between clinical symptoms and mortality, even after multivariate analysis.

3.3 Radiological findings

There is no specific radiological score for non-mucoviscidosis DDB. There are, however, many other scores for cystic fibrosis which have long been used for noncystic fibrosis. Among these scores, the modified Reiff score (41) is used

study the severity of dilatation (1=cylindrical; 2=moniliform; 3=cystic) the number of lobes affected. This score is simple and correlates with the severity of the disease, particularly colonisation by Pseudomonas Aeruginosa.
However, its main limitation remains the simplicity of this score, as shown by Loubeyre et al (29), that the prognosis of the disease depends on other radiological factors: the thickness of the bronchial wall, mucous plugs, mosaic perfusion and pulmonary emphysema.
Other scores have been used, such as the Bhalla score (42), which takes into account the presence of bullae, atelectasis, etc. This score was subsequently validated for non-mucoviscidosis DDB and correlated well with the prognosis of the disease. This score was subsequently validated for non-mucoviscidosis DDB and correlated well with the prognosis of the disease. The brody and robinson scores have not yet been validated in noncystic fibrosis DDB.
In our study, we did not use these radiological scores as we were interested in the FACED and BSI scores, which assess radiological factors such as the number of lobes for the two scores and the type of bronchiectasis (cystic) for the BSI.
No statistical relationship was found between disease severity and radiological features.

3.4 Microbiological elements

Colonisation with Pseudomonas Aeruginosa is associated with more severe COPD, a greater decline in FEV1 and higher mortality (31, 43). Several studies stress the importance of performing an ECBC in the stable state to search for pyocyanins with the aim of eradicating them (44). The impact of this germ on quality of life has also been demonstrated by Wilson et al (45).
In our work, contrary to the literature, no correlation was found between mortality and pyocyanin colonisation. The small number of colonised patients in our population may influence our results. On the other hand, although isolated in only 5 patients, superinfection by Moraxella catarrhalis was an independent risk factor for mortality after multivariate study.

3.5 Aetiologies

DDB is a heterogeneous disease, but its onset presupposes a combination of environmental factors, especially infectious ones, and a predisposing background. Variability between different continents has been widely incriminated, as illustrated in figure (27).
In the literature, based on a Chinese meta-analysis by YOUNG-HUA et al (46) and on a Spanish multicentre study (47), it has been estimated that infectious causes, including tuberculosis and infections at an early age, are the most common (30%), while LBD associated with chronic respiratory diseases is

found in 6.3% to 13.7% of cases. Pulmonary tuberculosis accounts for 18.6% of aetiologies in Spain.

In chronic respiratory diseases, the association of COPD and DDB is not uncommon, accounting for 3.9% to 7.8%. Moreover, this association has been considered a distinct phenotype, associated with frequent exacerbations, a fairly rich clinical picture and a poor prognosis. Among patients with severe COPD, an associated DDB is found in 30 to 50% of cases, and the prevalence of DDB increases with the severity of the COPD. In asthma, the association is less frequent (1.4 to 5.4%). Among severe or uncontrolled asthmatics, it is estimated that 20 to 30% have associated DDB. The causal relationship is as yet unknown. In these patients, the diagnosis of ABPA must be ruled out.

Other aetiologies include immune deficiency, which accounts for 59.4%, and to a lesser extent systemic diseases (1.4-3.8%), where rheumatoid arthritis has long been considered to be responsible for a poor prognosis, justifying close monitoring during medical check-ups in accordance with the BTS recommendations (48).

When all the aetiological investigations are negative, SBD is idiopathic, accounting for 24.2-44.8% of cases.

In Tunisia, there has been no study of the relationship between mortality and the aetiologies of DDB. Our results are not so different from the literature. Indeed, idiopathic DDB accounts for a large proportion in 65% of cases. The aetiologies we found were characterised by their variability, but none was correlated with mortality. On the other hand, COPD is associated with more severe DDB according to the BSI score, which is not the case if the FACED score is used.

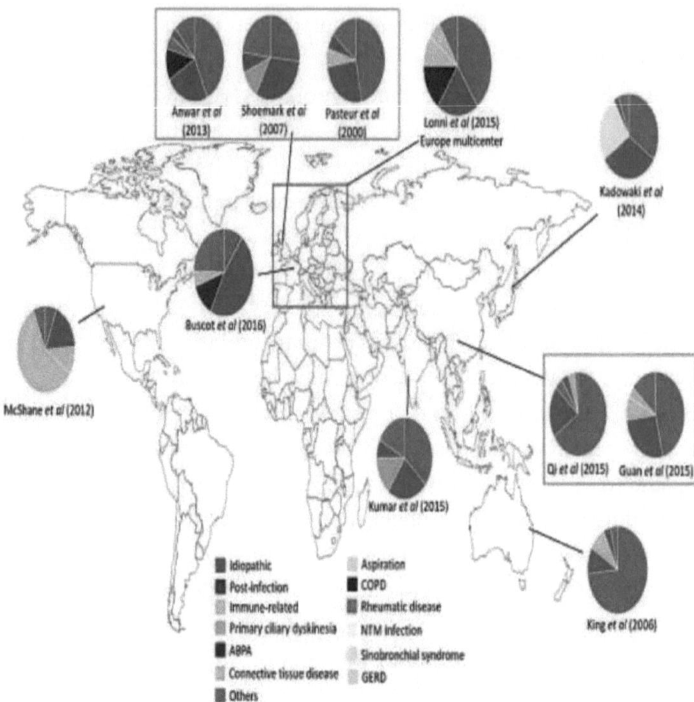

Chandrasekaran R et al Geographic variation in the aetiology, epidemiology and microbiology of bronchiectasis. BMC Pulm Med. Dec 2018

Figure 31: Etiologies of DDB worldwide by geographic and ethnic origin

4. Severity scores: BSI or FACED score?

To date, two severity scores have been validated for non-mucoviscidosis DDB: the FACED and the BSI . Both have advantages and disadvantages. The FACED score is easier to calculate and interpret because it contains 5 dichotomous variables. On the other hand, the BSI score is relatively complex, involving 9 non-dichotomous variables with precise values for each.

Both classify patients into 3 categories according to the degree of severity of the disease, with good prediction of mortality, but in different ways. The FACED was developed to predict 5-year mortality, whereas the BSI was developed not only to estimate mortality, but also to predict exacerbations, particularly those requiring hospitalisation, and to estimate quality of life.

Several studies have been carried out to compare the two scores in different populations. No studies have been carried out in Tunisia, despite the increase in the prevalence of the disease and in healthcare expenditure, especially during hospitalisation.

In a meta-analysis involving 7 European cohorts in 2016, Mac Donnel et al (10) compared the 2 scores on 1,612 patients. According to the authors, the 2 scores predict mortality, but the BSI is clearly superior in predicting exacerbations, quality of life, respiratory symptoms, physical exercise and decline in lung function.

A second study was also carried out in 2016 by Ellis et al (11) over 19 years of follow-up and studied the prediction of long-term mortality. At 5 years, the two scores provided a good prediction of mortality. At 15 years, both scores also predicted mortality, but with a better predictive value for the FACED score compared with the BSI. The weakness of this study was the small sample size (91 patients).

In 2017, a study by J.C Costa et al (49) compared the two scores. According to the authors, the BSI tends to classify patients mainly in the severe group and they explained these results by the higher number of variables in the BSI compared with the FACED. The weaknesses of this study are: the limited sample size (40 patients) and the fact that there were no deaths during the study, preventing the authors from studying mortality.

Edmundo et al (50) conducted a study in 2017 on a larger sample (198 patients) but with a different methodology. They divided the population into 2 categories: frequent exacerbators *(>2* exacerbations/year) and mild exacerbators (< exacerbations/year). They then studied the FACED and BSI scores in each category. Frequent exacerbators had risk factors such as older age, colonisation by Pseudomonas Aeruginosa, low FEV1 and Tiffneau ratio values and an association with COPD. On the other hand, if we look at the BSI and FACED scores, age and Pseudomonas Aeruginosa are the 2 factors involved in the frequency of exacerbations, and for the BSI we add the notion of hospitalisation and previous exacerbation.

4.1 Comparison by mortality prediction

According to our results, the BSI score is more sensitive in predicting mortality than the FACED score. The AUC values are different, with a significant AUC for the BSI score (0.77) but not significant for the FACED score (0.67).

Based on the BSI score, the Kaplein and Meyer survival curves show that 10-year survival is unfavourable, particularly for the severe group. On the other hand, survival is better for the mild to moderate group. In this case, the BSI is a good tool for distinguishing between patients who require fairly extensive treatment (severe group) and those who can be monitored by a family doctor (mild group). On the other hand, if we look at the Kaplein and Meyer curve for the FACED score, we find that mortality increases mainly in the moderate and severe groups. This discrepancy between the BSI and the FACED score is due to the difference in their variables and in the allocation of points for each variable. In fact, when analysing the mortality risk factors in our study, we found that certain factors were included in the BSI score and not in the FACED score, such as BMI, which may explain this discrepancy in the results for our population. Furthermore, when we look at the parameters making up the two scores, the values attributed to the same variable differ according to the score used. We were interested in the variables that constituted an independent risk factor for mortality, such as :

* **Age**: the BSI score takes into account 4 age groups, with values of 6 points above the age of 80, 4 points above the age of 70 and 2 points above the age of 50. These important values influence the total score, and age alone, rated at 6 points, already classifies moderate DDB. As for the FACED score, age over 70 years is worth 2 points and age scored at 2 points results in a classification of mild DDB. The same patient will therefore be classified differently depending on whether the BSI or FACED score is applied.

* **For exertional dyspnoea**: the classification was based essentially on the MRC for the BSI and mMRC for the FACED. The values attributed reach 3 points for stage 5 MRC for the BSI, but are lower for the FACED, reaching 1 point for stages 3 and 4 mMRC.

* **For FEV1**: the FACED score awards 2 points for any value <50%, whereas the BSI awards 3 points for FEV1 <30% and 1 point for FEV1 between 50 and 80%. FEV1, which is an independent mortality factor, is therefore underestimated by the FACED score, unlike the BSI.

4.2 Comparison by prediction of hospitalisations and exacerbations

Both scores were predictive of the risk hospitalisation, with an AUC >0.7 for each. In addition, the BSI score was more sensitive in predicting hospitalisations than the FACED score, since the corresponding AUC was 0.95 versus 0.69 for the FACED score (p<0.0001). In the literature, a CUA >0.8 is considered excellent, which is a strong point for the BSI. These results may be explained by the fact that the BSI score already includes hospitalisation in the previous 2 years among its variables. In addition, the BSI assigns 5 points to this variable, which immediately classifies the DDB as moderate. This value is considered to be overestimated if hospitalisation is excessive in certain specific cases (better access to care) whereas DDB is normally mild if this factor is not taken into account.

Neither score is a good predictor of exacerbations. Although the BSI takes this factor into account and awards 2 points for more than 3 exacerbations. Only 29% of patients are considered by the BSI to have had exacerbations exceeding 3/year. It is considered that a good questioning is necessary to detect the exact number of exacerbations since the patient can miss an exacerbation and thus modify the results of the BSI score. A score has been established by Martinez Garcia et al (51) called EXA-FACED to compensate for the FACED taking into account the exacerbation factor. This score has shown good predictive value for exacerbations and mortality.

4.3 Comparison by quality of life

DDB is a heterogeneous and fairly complex disease. As a result, the severity of this condition depends on an assessment of quality life. The SGRQ is a validated questionnaire that has long been used in chronic respiratory diseases such as COPD and DDB.

A meta-analysis by Spinou et al (52) in 2016 of 43 studies (3727 patients with DDB). The authors looked at the questionnaires used to estimate quality life in these patients. They concluded that the SGRQ is the most widely used (63%) and the most associated with exertional dyspnoea. However, this score is considered to be difficult for patients to complete over a long period of time. A more recent study in 2018 by Dudgeon et al (53) on a small sample (8 patients) concluded that the SGRQ had 3 negative points according to the participants: some questions were difficult, the questionnaire was not checked after 3 months and the true/false questions were not precise.

According to a 2013 study by Charrier et al (54), after 6 months of respiratory rehabilitation, they noted a significant improvement in patients' quality of life using the SGRQ score.

For our population, we calculated this questionnaire for survivors, and the results showed no difference between the two scores. Patients classified as severe had a total SGRQ of around 67 and 65 respectively for the BSI and FACED scores. No correlation was established between the scores and the SGRQ. The negative point of this questionnaire is the high number of parts (3 parts) and questions, which can be quite burdensome for the patient and the doctor to complete. Other questionnaires have been drawn up

4.4 Psychological status

Detecting anxiety-depressive disorders prove necessary in the overall management of a patient with DDB. As reported by Bousoffara et al (55) in a prospective Tunisian study conducted in 2014: the prevalence of depression was 20.8% and that of anxiety 22.7% using the HAD scale. The authors found that patients with anxiety disorders had more advanced exertional dyspnoea, low FEV1 and rapid progression to chronic respiratory failure. However, this study took into account patients without associated comorbidities, which is not the case in our study.

On the other hand, Olveira et al (56) studied the relationship and showed that symptoms of depression and anxiety are independent factors in patients' poor

quality of life.
In our study, 45 of 81 patients (55.6%) had an anxiety-depressive disorder.
The distribution of these patients differed according to the severity score used. If we used the FACED score, we would have 27 patients (60%) in the moderate group. On the other hand, using the BSI score, we would have 27 patients classified in the severe group.
The statistical relationship between the HAD scale and the 2 severity scores was significant, with p-values of around 0.004 and 0.039 for the FACED and BSI scores respectively.

Proposed new severity score for DDB :

Based on the results of the multivariate study, several risk factors for mortality were identified in our population. Some factors are not included in the BSI and FACED scores. Therefore, taking into account the BSI score which is the best applicable score for our population, we propose to take into account these identified risk factors: The number of comorbidities all kinds, a history of hypertension, asthma and GERD, socioeconomic status, superinfection by Branhamella Catarrhalis and non-use of Bromhexin.
According to the literature, systemic inflammation has been proposed as a potential explanation of the mechanism linking DDB, as in COPD, to co-morbidities, in part with the ageing process (57). Statins and macrolides have been shown to be effective in COPD in randomised controlled trials, due to their anti-inflammatory activity. The development of new selective anti-inflammatory drugs could be promising in the future (58). Furthermore, according to our work, Bromhexine plays a protective role, since the absence of this treatment presents an independent risk factor for mortality. Mucolytic treatment is routinely used, but a Cochrane review of the literature (59) reports that only 2 studies have looked at mycolytic agents in COPD, with or without exacerbations, but the results remain inconclusive.
Further studies will be needed to rate the new score items and validate them in the Tunisian population.

Table XXV: Variables making up the new score

Variable
Age (year)
<50
50-69
70-79
>80
Body mass index (BMI)
<18.5
>18.5

FEV1(%)
>80%
50-80%
30-49%
<30%

Hospitalisations in the previous 2 years
No
Yes

Exacerbations in the previous year 0-2
>3

Dyspnoea - MRC 1-3
4 5

Colonisation by Pseudomonas Aeruginosa No
Yes

Colonisation by another microorganism No
Yes

Radiological extension (> 3 lobes and/or cystic DDBs)
No Yes

Socioeconomic level Asthma

GERD
Number of co-morbidities

Superinfection by Branhamella Catarrhalis Non-use of Bromhexine

The strengths of our study are

The first strong point of this work is that it focuses on DDB, which is a neglected pathology, and demonstrates the high mortality associated with this condition.

On the other hand, we focused on the severity scores described in the literature (BSI and FACED) which have not previously been studied in the Tunisian population and this adds value to our work.

It should also be noted that the analysis of reliable and validated parameters such as the SGRQ, the HAD scale and the Charlson Comorbidity Index are strong points of this study.

Finally, the statistical analysis in this study made it possible to objectively compare the differences between the results.

Limitations of the study :

The first weakness of the study is the small sample size and the retrospective nature of the study.

For patients who had already died, the SGRQ did not estimate their quality of life, which led to a selection bias.

It should also be noted that the cytobacteriological examination of sputum is not systematic in our daily practice, especially in the stable state. This will reduce the likelihood of bacterial colonisation.

Conclusion

Diffuse bronchial dilatation (DDB) is an increasingly common condition in respiratory medicine. Today we are seeing more severe forms associated with increased mortality. Diagnosis of diffuse bronchial dilatation is easily established using multi-bar CT scans, but the aetiological and therapeutic approach can be difficult, mainly due to the heterogeneous nature of the disease.

This is why we thought it would be interesting to contribute, through this retrospective study of 110 cases of patients collected between 2009 and 2018 in the pneumology unit of the Hédi Chaker Hospital in Sfax, to analysing the prognostic factors and comparing the two severity scores, BSI and FACED, with the aim of choosing the best one for our population.

Our results are as follows:

Demographic data showed a sex ratio of 1.4 with a male predominance (58%). The mean age was 60 years. Smoking was present in 46% of patients.

Personal history was variable, dominated by cardiovascular comorbidities, GERD, asthma and COPD. Socioeconomic status was average in almost half the cases.

The clinical picture remains dominated by exertional dyspnoea, followed by productive cough and morning bronchorrhoea.

Chest CT confirms the diagnosis of DDB and studies the type of lesions. In our population, cylindrical forms are the most common (75%) and associations between the different types are not uncommon (51.9%).

A microbiological study using ECBC showed 5 patients colonised by pyocyanins. On the other hand, superinfections are not uncommon, such as pyocyanus, which affected 24 patients, and other germs were present in 22 cases.

Spirometry was used to measure FEV1, which averaged 52%. The frequency of obstructive ventilatory disorder was also noted in 45% of cases.

The aetiologies of DDB in our population are mainly infectious, including tuberculosis (19%) and infections in young people (9%), while systemic diseases are less common (7%). In the majority of cases, DDB remains idiopathic (65%).

Prognosis:

Mortality in our population is high, at 20.6%. It increases with age, reaching 13.7% over the age of 65. It is predominantly male (25.9%) with no significant relationship. Data in the literature is limited, as this is still an under-diagnosed condition. In the United Kingdom, mortality is high, reaching 29%. Other studies have shown significant mortality linked to DDB, notably in Turkey (16.3%), Belgium (10.6%) and South Korea (2.9% in hospital).

The data from our study point to numerous independent risk factors for mortality, which can be summarised as follows:

- Medium to high socio-economic level
- The number of co-morbidities
- Certain antecedents: High blood pressure, asthma, GERD
- Superinfection by Branhamella Catarrhalis
- Not using Bromhexine
- Hospitalisations / previous 2 years

Concerning severity scores: BSI versus FACED

For our population, the BSI score is better at predicting long-term mortality. In addition, it is more sensitive in predicting hospital admissions, which is already an independent risk factor for mortality.

Similarly, the BSI score had a statistically significant relationship with the decline in FEV1. On the other hand, no score was able to predict exacerbations in our series. These results are expected, since in the literature the BSI score is considered by most studies to be sensitive in mortality as well as in predicting exacerbations, hospitalisations, decline in FEV1 and impairment of quality of life.

At present, quality of life is an essential factor in assessing the severity of DDB. The SGRQ reflects quality of life in our patients, with a significant relationship with the HAD scale, the number of exacerbations and hospitalisations.

Bibliography

1. Fuschillo S, De Felice A, Balzano G. Mucosal inflammation in idiopathic bronchiectasis: cellular and molecular mechanisms. Eur Respir J. 1 Feb 2008;31(2):396- 406.
2. Quint JK, Millett ERC, Joshi M, Navaratnam V, Thomas SL, Hurst JR, et al. Changes in the incidence, prevalence and mortality of bronchiectasis in the UK from 2004 to 2013: a population-based cohort study. Eur Respir J. Jan 2016;47(1):186- 93.
3. Goeminne PC, Hernandez F, Diel R, Filonenko A, Hughes R, Juelich F, et al. The economic burden of bronchiectasis - known and unknown: a systematic review. BMC Pulm Med. Dec 2019;19(1):54.
4. King PT, Holdsworth SR, Freezer NJ, Villanueva E, Holmes PW. Characterisation of the onset and presenting clinical features of adult bronchiectasis. Respir Med. Dec 2006;100(12):2183- 9.
5. Loebinger MR, Wells AU, Hansell DM, Chinyanganya N, Devaraj A, Meister M, et al. Mortality in bronchiectasis: a long-term study assessing the factors influencing survival. Eur Respir J. 1 Oct 2009;34(4):843- 9.
6. Martínez-García MA, Perpiñá-Tordera M, Román-Sánchez P, Soler-Cataluña JJ. Quality-of-Life Determinants in Patients With Clinically Stable Bronchiectasis. Chest. August 2005;128(2):739- 45.
7. Chalmers JD, Goeminne P, Aliberti S, McDonnell MJ, Lonni S, Davidson J, et al. The Bronchiectasis Severity Index. An International Derivation and Validation Study. Am J Respir Crit Care Med. March 2014;189(5):576- 85.
8. Martinez-Garcia MA, de Gracia J, Vendrell Relat M, Giron R-M, Maiz Carro L, de la Rosa Carrillo D, et al. Multidimensional approach to non-cystic fibrosis bronchiectasis: the FACED score. Eur Respir J. 1 May 2014;43(5):1357- 67.
9. Athanazio R, Pereira MC, Gramblicka G, Cavalcanti-Lundgren F, de Figueiredo MF, Arancibia F, et al. Latin America validation of FACED score in patients with bronchiectasis: an analysis of six cohorts. BMC Pulm Med. Dec 2017;17(1):73.
10. McDonnell MJ, Aliberti S, Goeminne PC, Dimakou K, Zucchetti SC, Davidson J, et al. Multidimensional severity assessment in bronchiectasis: an analysis of seven European cohorts. Thorax. Dec 2016;71(12):1110- 8.
11. Ellis HC, Cowman S, Fernandes M, Wilson R, Loebinger MR. Predicting mortality in bronchiectasis using bronchiectasis severity index and FACED scores: a 19-year cohort study. Eur Respir J. Feb 2016;47(2):482- 9.
12. Onen ZP, Eris Gulbay B, Sen E, Akkoca Yildiz Ö, Saryal S, Acican T, et al. Analysis of the factors related to mortality in patients with bronchiectasis. Respir Med. Jul 2007;101(7):1390- 7.
13. Minov J, Karadzinska-Bislimovska J, Vasilevska K, Stoleski S, Mijakoski D. Assessment of the Non-Cystic Fibrosis Bronchiectasis Severity: The FACED Score vs the Bronchiectasis Severity Index. Open Respir Med J. March 31, 2015;9(1):46- 51.
14. Martínez-García MÁ, Máiz L, Olveira C, Girón RM, de la Rosa D, Blanco M, et al. Spanish Guidelines on the Evaluation and Diagnosis of Bronchiectasis in Adults. Arch Bronconeumol Engl Ed. Feb 2018;54(2):79- 87.
15. Charlson ME, Pompei P, Ales KL, MacKenzie CR. A new method of classifying prognostic comorbidity in longitudinal studies: Development and validation. J Chronic Dis. Jan 1987;40(5):373- 83.
16. Jones PW, Quirk FH, Baveystock CM. The St George's Respiratory Questionnaire. Respir Med. Sept 1991;85:25- 31.
17. Martínez García MA, Perpiñá Tordera M, Román Sánchez P, Cataluña S. Internal Consistency and Validity of the Spanish Version of the St. George' Respiratory Questionnaire for Use in Patients With Clinically Stable Bronchiectasis. Arch Bronconeumol Engl Ed. March 2005;41(3):110- 7.
18. Ringshausen FC, de Roux A, Pletz MW, Hämäläinen N, Welte T, Rademacher J. Bronchiectasis-

Associated Hospitalizations in Germany, 2005-2011: A Population-Based Study of Disease Burden and Trends. Fessler MB, editor. PLoS ONE. 1 Aug 2013;8(8):e71109.
19. Seitz AE, Olivier KN, Steiner CA, Montes de Oca R, Holland SM, Prevots DR. Trends and Burden of Bronchiectasis-Associated Hospitalizations in the United States, 1993-2006. Chest. Oct 2010;138(4):944- 9.
20. Choi H, Yang B, Nam H, Kyoung D-S, Sim YS, Park HY, et al. Population-based prevalence of bronchiectasis and associated comorbidities in South Korea. Eur Respir J. Aug 2019;54(2):1900194.
21. Aksamit TR, O'Donnell AE, Barker A, Olivier KN, Winthrop KL, Daniels MLA, et al. Adult Patients With Bronchiectasis. Chest. May 2017;151(5):982- 92.
22. Sadighi Akha AA. Aging and the immune system: An overview. J Immunol Methods. dec 2018;463:21- 6.
23. Field CE. Bronchiectasis. Third report on a follow-up study of medical and surgical cases from childhood. Arch Dis Child. 1 Oct 1969;44(237):551- 61.
24. King P. The pathophysiology of bronchiectasis. Int J Chron Obstruct Pulmon Dis. Oct 2009;411.
25. Lonni S, Chalmers JD, Goeminne PC, McDonnell MJ, Dimakou K, De Soyza A, et al. Etiology of Non-Cystic Fibrosis Bronchiectasis in Adults and Its Correlation to Disease Severity. Ann Am Thorac Soc. Dec 2015;12(12):1764- 70.
26. Lee AL, Button BM, Denehy L, Wilson JW. Gastro-Oesophageal Reflux in Noncystic Fibrosis Bronchiectasis. Pulm Med. 2011;2011:1- 6.
27. Chandrasekaran R, Mac Aogáin M, Chalmers JD, Elborn SJ, Chotirmall SH. Geographic variation in the aetiology, epidemiology and microbiology of bronchiectasis. BMC Pulm Med. Dec 2018;18(1):83.
28. Lynch DA, Newell J, Hale V, Dyer D, Corkery K, Fox NL, et al. Correlation of CT findings with clinical evaluations in 261 patients with symptomatic bronchiectasis. Am J Roentgenol. July 1999;173(1):53- 8.
29. Loubeyre P, Paret M, Revel D, Wiesendanger T, Brune J. Thin-Section CT Detection of Emphysema Associated With Bronchiectasis and Correlation With Pulmonary Function Tests. Chest. Feb 1996;109(2):360- 5.
30. Amorim A, Meira L, Redondo M, Ribeiro M, Castro R, Rodrigues M, et al. Chronic Bacterial Infection Prevalence, Risk Factors, and Characteristics: A Bronchiectasis Population-Based Prospective Study. J Clin Med. March 6, 2019;8(3):315.
31. Finch S, McDonnell MJ, Abo-Leyah H, Aliberti S, Chalmers JD. A Comprehensive Analysis of the Impact of *Pseudomonas aeruginosa* Colonisation on Prognosis in Adult Bronchiectasis. Ann Am Thorac Soc. 10 Sep 2015;AnnalsATS.201506-333OC.
32. Machado BC, Jacques PS, Penteado LP, Roth Dalcin P de T. Prognostic Factors in Adult Patients with Non-Cystic Fibrosis Bronchiectasis. Lung. Dec 2018;196(6):691- 7.
33. Goeminne P, Scheers H, Decraene A, Seys S, Dupont L. Risk factors for morbidity and death in non-cystic fibrosis bronchiectasis: a retrospective cross-sectional analysis of CT diagnosed bronchiectatic patients. Respir Res. 2012;13(1):21.
34. Poppelwell L, Chalmers JD. Defining severity in non-cystic fibrosis bronchiectasis. Expert Rev Respir Med. Apr 2014;8(2):249- 62.
35. McDonnell MJ, Aliberti S, Goeminne PC, Restrepo MI, Finch S, Pesci A, et al. Comorbidities and the risk of mortality in patients with bronchiectasis: an international multicentre cohort study. Lancet Respir Med. Dec 2016;4(12):969- 79.
36. Martinez-Garcia MA, Miravitlles M. Bronchiectasis in COPD patients: more than a comorbidity? Int J Chron Obstruct Pulmon Dis. May 2017;Volume 12:1401- 11.
37. Labaki WW, Han MK. Impact of bronchiectasis on the frequency and severity of respiratory exacerbations in COPD. Int J Chron Obstruct Pulmon Dis. Jul 2018;Volume 13:2335- 8.
38. Mandal P, Morice AH, Chalmers JD, Hill AT. Symptoms of airway reflux predict exacerbations and quality of life in bronchiectasis. Respir Med. Jul 2013;107(7):1008- 13.

39. McDonnell MJ, O'Toole D, Ward C, Pearson JP, Lordan JL, De Soyza A, et al. A qualitative synthesis of gastro-oesophageal reflux in bronchiectasis: Current understanding and future risk. Respir Med. August 2018;141:132- 43.
40. Murray MP, Pentland JL, Turnbull K, MacQuarrie S, Hill AT. Sputum colour: a useful clinical tool in non-cystic fibrosis bronchiectasis. Eur Respir J. 1 August 2009;34(2):361- 4.
41. Reiff DB, Wells AU, Carr DH, Cole PJ, Hansell DM. CT findings in bronchiectasis: limited value in distinguishing between idiopathic and specific types. Am J Roentgenol. August 1995;165(2):261- 7.
42. Park J, Kim S, Lee YJ, Park JS, Cho Y-J, Yoon HI, et al. Factors associated with radiologic progression of non-cystic fibrosis bronchiectasis during long-term follow-up: Radiologic progression of bronchiectasis. Respirology. august 2016;21(6):1049- 54.
43. McDonnell MJ, Jary HR, Perry A, MacFarlane JG, Hester KLM, Small T, et al. Non cystic fibrosis bronchiectasis: A longitudinal retrospective observational cohort study of Pseudomonas persistence and resistance. Respir Med. June 2015;109(6):716- 26.
44. Tassart G, Pieters T, Gohy S. MANAGEMENT OF ADULT BRONCHIECTASIS. Rev Med Liege. :9.
45. Wilson CB, Jones PW, O'Leary CJ, Hansell DM, Cole PJ, Wilson R. Effect of sputum bacteriology on the quality of life of patients with bronchiectasis. Eur Respir J. 1 Aug 1997;10(8):1754- 60.
46. Gao Y, Guan W, Liu S, Wang L, Cui J, Chen R, et al. Aetiology of bronchiectasis in adults: A systematic literature review: Aetiology in bronchiectasis. Respirology. nov 2016;21(8):1376- 83.
47. Olveira C, Padilla A, Martínez-García M-Á, de la Rosa D, Girón R-M, Vendrell M, et al. Etiology of Bronchiectasis in a Cohort of 2047 Patients. An Analysis of the Spanish Historical Bronchiectasis Registry. Arch Bronconeumol Engl Ed. Jul 2017;53(7):366- 74.
48. T Hill A, L Sullivan A, D Chalmers J, De Soyza A, Stuart Elborn J, Andres Floto R, et al. British Thoracic Society Guideline for bronchiectasis in adults. Thorax. Jan 2019;74(Suppl 1):1- 69.
49. Costa JC, Machado JN, Ferreira C, Gama J, Rodrigues C. The Bronchiectasis Severity Index and FACED score for assessment of the severity of bronchiectasis. Pulmonology. May 2018;24(3):149- 54.
50. Rosales-Mayor E, Polverino E, Raguer L, Alcaraz V, Gabarrus A, Ranzani O, et al. Comparison of two prognostic scores (BSI and FACED) in a Spanish cohort of adult patients with bronchiectasis and improvement of the FACED predictive capacity for exacerbations. Loukides S, editor. PLOS ONE. 6 Apr 2017;12(4):e0175171.
51. Martinez-Garcia MA, Athanazio RA, Girón RM, Máiz-Carro L, de la Rosa D, Olveira C, et al. Predicting high risk of exacerbations in bronchiectasis: the E-FACED score. Int J Chron Obstruct Pulmon Dis. Jan 2017;Volume 12:275- 84.
52. Spinou A, Fragkos KC, Lee KK, Elston C, Siegert RJ, Loebinger MR, et al. The validity of health-related quality of life questionnaires in bronchiectasis: a systematic review and metaanalysis. Thorax. August 2016;71(8):683- 94.
53. Dudgeon EK, Crichton M, Chalmers JD. 'The missing ingredient': the patient perspective of health related quality of life in bronchiectasis: a qualitative study. BMC Pulm Med. Dec 2018;18(1):81.
54. Charrier M. Respiratory rehabilitation and quality of life in patients with bronchial dilatation. 2013;56.
55. Boussoffara L, Boudawara N, Gharsallaoui Z, Sakka M, Knani J. Anxiodepressive disorders and bronchial dilatation. Rev Mal Respir. March 2014;31(3):230- 6.
56. Olveira C, Olveira G, Gaspar I, Dorado A, Cruz I, Soriguer F, et al. Depression and anxiety symptoms in bronchiectasis: associations with health-related quality of life. Qual Life Res. Apr 2013;22(3):597- 605.
57. Fabbri LM, Luppi F, Beghe B, Rabe KF. Complex chronic comorbidities of COPD. Eur Respir J.

1 Jan 2008;31(1):204- 12.
58. Koser U, Hill A. What's new in the management of adult bronchiectasis? F1000Research. 20 Apr 2017;6:527.
59. Welsh EJ, Evans DJ, Fowler SJ, Spencer S. Interventions for bronchiectasis: an overview of Cochrane systematic reviews. Cochrane Airways Group, editor. Cochrane Database Syst Rev [Internet]. 2015 Jul 14 [cited 2019 Dec 30]; Available from: http://doi.wiley.com/10.1002/14651858.CD010337.pub2

Appendix 1: Data collection form

Last name First name File no.

Age

Gender

BMI

Rural origin Urban

Profession

<u>Habits</u>

Active / passive smoking Number of PA

Alcohol

<u>ATCD</u>

Obesity

Diabetes

COPD

Asthma measles

GERD

HTA

Heart disease: ischaemic / rhythm disorders

Neoplastic

Measles

Number of exacerbations in the previous year :

Number of hospitalisations during the previous 2 years :

<u>Symptoms</u>

Dyspnoea on exertion: mMRC/MRC stage

Haemoptysis : abundance recurrence

Cough : dry productive

Morning bronchorrhoea

Chest pain : type

Recurrent lower respiratory infections

<u>Spirometry</u>

FEV1 (%)

FEV1/FVC(%)

CVL (%)

<u>ECBC</u>

History of infection with Pseudomonas Aéruginosa :

Colonisation by Pseudomonas Aéruginosa

Other germs: specify

Chest CT scan

Number of lobes :

Type of lesions :

Cylindrical / moniliform / cystic

ADP : Mediastinal / hilar

Pleuresis

Emphysema

Quality of life assessment

Saint George questionnaire (SGRQ)

Etiology of the disease

Tuberculosis

Pneumonia at an early age Idiopathic systemic disease

Other

Treatment

Inhaled corticoids

Systemic corticoids

Inhaled antibotics

LAMA

LABA

Theophylline

Bissolvan

Surgery: lobectomy / segmentectomy / pneumonectomy

Death / time between diagnosis and death

Severity scores BSI score FACED score

Appendix 2: Charlson comorbidity index

Items	Weighting	Score
Myocardial infarction	1 point	
Congestive heart failure	1 point	
Peripheral vascular diseases	1 point	
Cerebrovascular diseases (except hemiplegia)	1 point	
Dementia	1 point	
Chronic lung diseases	1 point	
Connective tissue diseases	1 point	
Oesogastro-duodenal ulcers	1 point	
Uncomplicated diabetes	1 point	
Mild liver disease	1 point	
Hemiplegia	2 points	
Moderate or severe kidney disease	2 points	
Diabetes with target organ damage	2 points	
Cancer	2 points	
Leukaemia	2 points	
Lymphoma	2 points	
Multiple myeloma	2 points	
Moderate or severe liver disease	3 points	
Metastatic tumour	6 points	
AIDS	6 points	

Appendix 3: FACED score

Items	Points
Chronic colonisation by Pseudomonas Aeruginosa	
No	0
Yes	1
Dyspnoea mMRC score	
0-II	0
III-IV	1
FEV1 % predicted	
>50%	0
<50%	2
Age	
<70 years	0
>70 years	2
Number of lobes	
1-2	0
>2	1

Points	Score
0-2	DDB light
3-4	Moderate DDB
5-7	Severe DDB

Appendix 4: BSI score

Variable Points	
Age (years) <50	0
50-69	2
70-79	4
>80	6
Body Mass Index (BMI) <18.5	0
>18.5	2
FEV1(%)	
>80%	0
50-80%	1
30-49%	2
<30%	3
Hospitalisations in the previous 2 years No	0
Yes	5
Exacerbations in the previous year 0-2	0
>3	2
Dyspnoea - MRC 1-3	0
4	2
5	3
Colonisation by Pseudomonas Aeruginosa No	0
Yes	3
Colonisation by another microorganism No	0
Yes	1
Radiological extension (> 3 lobes and/or cystic DDBs) **No** **Yes**	0 1

Points	Score
0-4	low BSI score
5-8	BSI intermediate score
> 9	BSI high score

Appendix 5: HAH scale

Outil associé à la recommandation de bonne pratique « Arrêt de la consommation de tabac : du dépistage individuel au maintien de l'abstinence »

Échelle HAD : *Hospital Anxiety and Depression scale*

L'échelle HAD est un instrument qui permet de dépister les troubles anxieux et dépressifs. Elle comporte 14 items cotés de 0 à 3. Sept questions se rapportent à l'anxiété (total A) et sept autres à la dimension dépressive (total D), permettant ainsi l'obtention de deux scores (note maximale de chaque score = 21).

1. Je me sens tendu(e) ou énervé(e)
- La plupart du temps 3
- Souvent 2
- De temps en temps 1
- Jamais 0

2. Je prends plaisir aux mêmes choses qu'autrefois
- Oui, tout autant 0
- Pas autant 1
- Un peu seulement 2
- Presque plus 3

3. J'ai une sensation de peur comme si quelque chose d'horrible allait m'arriver
- Oui, très nettement 3
- Oui, mais ce n'est pas trop grave 2
- Un peu, mais cela ne m'inquiète pas 1
- Pas du tout 0

4. Je ris facilement et vois le bon côté des choses
- Autant que par le passé 0
- Plus autant qu'avant 1
- Vraiment moins qu'avant 2
- Plus du tout 3

5. Je me fais du souci
- Très souvent 3
- Assez souvent 2
- Occasionnellement 1
- Très occasionnellement 0

6. Je suis de bonne humeur
- Jamais 3
- Rarement 2
- Assez souvent 1
- La plupart du temps 0

7. Je peux rester tranquillement assis(e) à ne rien faire et me sentir décontracté(e)
- Oui, quoi qu'il arrive 0
- Oui, en général 1
- Rarement 2
- Jamais 3

8. J'ai l'impression de fonctionner au ralenti
- Presque toujours 3
- Très souvent 2
- Parfois 1
- Jamais 0

9. J'éprouve des sensations de peur et j'ai l'estomac noué
- Jamais 0
- Parfois 1
- Assez souvent 2
- Très souvent 3

10. Je ne m'intéresse plus à mon apparence
- Plus du tout 3
- Je n'y accorde pas autant d'attention que je devrais 2
- Il se peut que je n'y fasse plus autant attention 1
- J'y prête autant d'attention que par le passé 0

11. J'ai la bougeotte et n'arrive pas à tenir en place
- Oui, c'est tout à fait le cas 3
- Un peu 2
- Pas tellement 1
- Pas du tout 0

12. Je me réjouis d'avance à l'idée de faire certaines choses
- Autant qu'avant 0
- Un peu moins qu'avant 1
- Bien moins qu'avant 2
- Presque jamais 3

13. J'éprouve des sensations soudaines de panique
- Vraiment très souvent 3
- Assez souvent 2
- Pas très souvent 1
- Jamais 0

14. Je peux prendre plaisir à un bon livre ou à une bonne émission de radio ou de télévision
- Souvent 0
- Parfois 1
- Rarement 2
- Très rarement 3

Scores

Additionnez les points des réponses : 1, 3, 5, 7, 9, 11, 13 : Total A = ______

Additionnez les points des réponses : 2, 4, 6, 8, 10, 12, 14 : Total D = ______

Interprétation

Pour dépister des symptomatologies anxieuses et dépressives, l'interprétation suivante peut être proposée pour chacun des scores (A et D) :

- 7 ou moins : absence de symptomatologie
- 8 à 10 : symptomatologie douteuse – 11 et plus : symptomatologie certaine.

Selon les résultats, il sera peut-être nécessaire de demander un avis spécialisé.

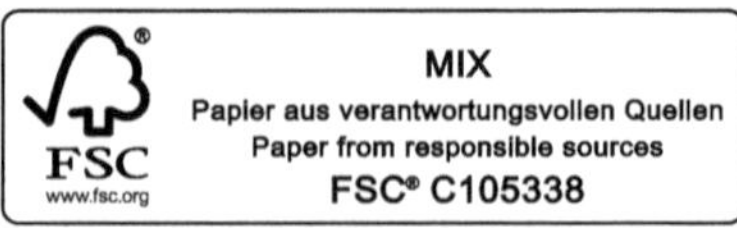

Printed by Books on Demand GmbH, Norderstedt / Germany